Pauline Wills runs a thriving practice in reflexology and colour therapy in London. She also gives talks and workshops throughout Europe and runs the Oracle School of Colour. This school runs an accredited two-year course for colour practitioners and certificated courses for qualified reflexologists who wish to combine colour with reflexology.

Reflexology and Color Therapy

A PRACTICAL INTRODUCTION

*Combining the healing benefits of
two complementary therapies*

Pauline Wills

ELEMENT

Shaftesbury, Dorset ● Boston, Massachusetts
Melbourne, Victoria

© Element Books Limited 1998
Text © Pauline Wills 1992, 1998

First published as *The Reflexology & Colour Therapy Workbook*
in the UK in 1992 by Element Books Limited

This revised edition first published in the US in 1998 by
Element Books, Inc.
160 North Washington Street,
Boston, MA 02114

Published in the UK in 1988 by Element Books Limited
Shaftesbury, Dorset SP7 8BP

Published in Australia in 1998 by Element Books and distributed by
Penguin Australia Limited
487 Maroondah Highway, Ringwood, Victoria 3134

Cover design by Slatter-Anderson
Designed by Linda Reed and Associates
Printed and bound in Great Britain by
Butler & Tanner Ltd., Frome and London

Library of Congress Cataloging in Publication Data available

ISBN 1-86204 399 X

This book is dedicated to Patricia and Christopher Jackson for all the love, support and encouragement that they have given to me during a very difficult time in my life.

Thank you

Contents

Introduction

My first appreciation of colour arose about twenty-eight years ago when I started to study and practise yoga. During this time, I learnt about the subtle anatomy and the colours which penetrate this, appearing as a continually changing rainbow. I became fascinated with colour and when I started to teach yoga, I taught my students how to visualize colour with postures to enhance and bring about a greater therapeutic effect.

Whilst teaching yoga, I began to study reflexology and learnt that the soles of both feet and the palms of both hands are mirror images of the physical body. Terminating on the soles of the feet and palms of the hands are the ten energy channels which run through the body. If these channels become blocked, energy is unable to flow to the various organs and muscles, thus creating dis-ease in the physical body. I was taught that by using certain pressure techniques on the zones of the feet or hands, these blockages can be released, allowing the energy to flow freely thus bringing the body back into harmony. When I qualified and started to practise this complementary therapy, I realized that one is not only working with the physical body but also with the aura or subtle anatomy. Again I came into contact with colour. I was by now fascinated with colour and decided that I wanted to learn more about it.

Quite by chance (if anything that happens is by chance) a colleague saw a notice in her local library advertising a course in colour and colour healing, run by Lily Cornford of the Maitreya School of Healing. Here I started to learn about the colours, their vibrational frequencies and how they were used in healing. I learnt to sensitize my physical body to feel and to visualize colour and then how to channel these colours through me for healing. It was a wonderful experience.

Some time after completing this course, whilst visiting an exhibition, I discovered the Hygeia College of Colour Therapy, run by Theo Gimbel. I enrolled for his course and after two years qualified as a colour therapist. I then continued to study in order to sit for the diploma in colour therapy which enabled me to teach it.

Working as a colour therapist and reflexologist, I started to combine the two. Firstly I carried out a normal reflexology treatment and then I put colour into the zones which were painful, denoting energy blocks. I was greatly rewarded because the results were excellent. I administered colour into the zones by visualizing the appropriate colour being channelled through me, into my fingers and into the patient. On reflecting upon how other reflexologists could use colour, I realized that some may have difficulty with this method, so I devised what is now known as the Reflexology Crystal Torch.

This instrument shines light through stained glass discs into a small single-terminated crystal. The crystal is set into copper in which a space is provided for the stained glass disc. Copper is related to the planet Venus, the planet of love; thereby, colour is brought into the crystal through the medium of love. Stained glass is always used in preference to gels, because it contains the full vibrational spectrum of each colour. This enables the patient to absorb the exact shade that he or she needs. Gels are static in that they contain just one vibration and if a patient does not require that particular shade or vibration, then it has little or no effect.

I have been working with the Reflexology Crystal Torch for just over eight years and have seen some excellent results. For example, tinnitus, which can be very difficult to treat, has responded well. One very nervous patient asked me, when I applied blue to the solar plexus reflex, if I had ever been given a pre-med. I said that I had, many years ago. She said she felt as if I had just given her one, and that she felt very sleepy and relaxed. Another patient commented that he could feel the vibrations travelling through his leg, into his body. He said that when the vibrations stopped, he felt as though a huge weight had been removed from his abdomen.

I hope that anyone who reads this book and starts to use colour with reflexology will have the same wonderful results that I have had.

Pauline Wills

CHAPTER 1

Electromagnetic Energy

The electromagnetic energy spectrum ranges from the longest energy waves, namely radio waves, to the shortest energy waves which are the cosmic rays. In between these two come infra-red rays, visible light, ultra violet light, X-rays and gamma rays. This complete spectrum contains sixty or seventy octaves and all the electromagnetic energy travels at about 186,000 miles per second. (See Figure 1.)

Starting with the longest energy waves and working up the scale to the shortest energy waves, let us look at some of the properties of these rays and how they are being used scientifically and in medicine.

The longest electromagnetic waves, radio waves, include commercial broadcasting, short-wave bands and FM radio, television and radar.

Radio waves are used for 'wireless', trans-oceanic communication and ship-to-shore communication. They are also used in industry to raise the temperature of metals for hardening purposes.

The commercial broadcasting rays have the ability of bouncing back from the ionosphere and travelling round the earth.

Short-wave bands are used for distance broadcasting by police, ships and sometimes amateurs. Diathermy, which is the application of electric currents to produce heat in the deeper tissues of the body, uses these electromagnetic waves. This is achieved by strapping electrodes, through which the heat is generated, to specific parts of the body. This treatment is used for the relief of rheumatism, arthritis and neuralgia.

Unlike commercial broadcasting rays, FM radio, television and radar waves penetrate the ionosphere and are not reflected back. They follow a straight path, necessitating their direction to be controlled.

Next we come to the infra-red waves. These include photographic and radiant heat waves. The infra-red rays are invisible but have the power to travel great distances and to penetrate heavy atmospheres. Photographic plates are sensitive to these rays, therefore they can be used to take pictures which the human eye has difficulty in seeing. Radiant heat waves are used for heating and drying purposes. They can be emitted by steam radiators, electric heaters and infra-red lamps.

Next comes visible light. As well as the colours of the spectrum, science also includes infra-red and ultraviolet light under this section. Visible light rays are said to measure about 1/33,000 of an inch at the red end of the spectrum and about 1/67,000 of an inch at the violet end. These rays will be discussed in Chapter 7.

Moving up the scale, we come to the ultraviolet light. This encompasses fluorescent and erythemal rays. The longest waves of ultraviolet radiation produce fluorescent light. Even though widely used, it has been shown that this type of lighting can be very detrimental to health. For further information on this, read *Healing Through Colour* by Theo Gimbel. Under ultraviolet light, certain substances become luminous; for example, butter glows yellow and margarine glows blue. Cancer tissue glows a vivid yellow and live teeth glow, whereas dead teeth do not. This phenomenon has been beneficially used by science and medicine.

The erythemal rays are responsible for producing a suntan. They are also used for the synthetic production of vitamin D.

As the wave lengths become shorter, we come to the X-rays. These include grenz rays (which are soft X-rays) and hard X-rays. 'Hard X-rays' are those which destroy the cells of the physical body, ie those used in the treatment of malignant tumours. 'Soft X-rays' are those which do minimal damage and are used for X-raying the physical body. X-rays are widely used by the medical profession for diagnostic purposes. Even though they are invaluable for this purpose, overdoses can cause serious damage such as anaemia, roentgen sickness and carcinomas. If used during pregnancy, they can cause serious deformities to the foetus.

The hard X-rays are used medically for deep-seated afflictions and by industry to detect flaws in metal.

Nearing the end of the scale are the gamma or radium rays. These were discovered by Pierre and Marie Curie at the beginning of the twentieth century. These are specially penetrating rays, emitted by a

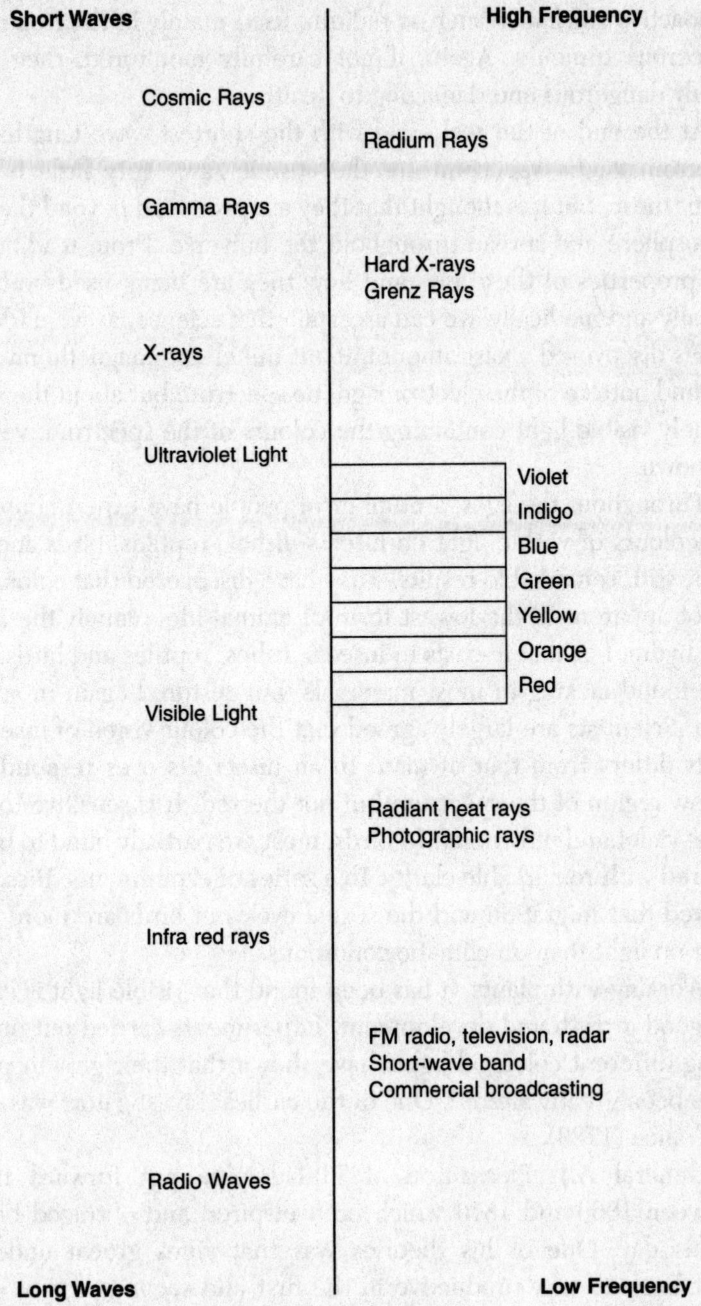

Short Waves   **High Frequency**

Cosmic Rays

Radium Rays

Gamma Rays

Hard X-rays
Grenz Rays

X-rays

Ultraviolet Light

	Violet
	Indigo
	Blue
	Green
	Yellow
	Orange
	Red

Visible Light

Radiant heat rays
Photographic rays

Infra red rays

FM radio, television, radar
Short-wave band
Commercial broadcasting

Radio Waves

Long Waves   **Low Frequency**

Fig. 1 The electromagnetic spectrum

radioactive substance such as radium, used mainly in the treatment of cancerous tumours. Again, if not carefully monitored, they can be highly dangerous and damaging to health.

At the end of the scale and with the shortest wave lengths in the electromagnetic spectrum are the cosmic rays. Very little is known about these, but it is thought that they are produced beyond the earth's atmosphere and spread throughout the universe. From reading about the properties of these rays and how they are being used both scientifically and medically, we can ascertain that science, as we understand it, has discovered a vast amount about the electromagnetic rays at the top and bottom of the electromagnetic spectrum but about the middle, namely visible light containing the colours of the spectrum, very little is known.

Throughout the ages, a number of people have experimented with the colours of visible light on insects, fishes, reptiles, birds and mammals, with remarkable results. They have discovered that colour vision is not apparent in the lowest form of animal life, namely the amoeba and hydra, but that it exists in insects, fishes, reptiles and birds. Again, it is found lacking in most mammals, but restored again in apes and man. Scientists are largely agreed that the colour vision of insects and birds differs from that of man. In an insect, its eyes respond to the yellow region of the spectrum but not the red. It is sensitive to green, blue, violet and ultraviolet. In birds, most are partially blind to blue but see red with remarkable clarity. In a series of experiments, Bissonnette proved that migration and the sexual cycles in birds are more dependent on light than on climatic conditions.

Working with plants, it has been found that visible light is essential for good growth and development. Experiments carried out on plants using different coloured lights have shown that their growth patterns have been greatly altered. One of the earliest investigators was Ressier of France (1783).

General A.J. Pleasanton of Philadelphia put forward theories between 1860 and 1870 which both inspired and outraged botanists of his day. One of his theories was that vines grown under blue light became very productive in the first and second year of growth, whereas under normal light they would take five or six years to reach the same stage of production. In 1895, C. Flammarion claimed that plants flourished under red light. He said that this colour produced taller plants with thinner leaves. Under blue light, he stated that the plant was weak and underdeveloped. Other investigators such as L.C. Corbett (1902), Fritz Schanz (1918), H.W. Popp (1926) and S. Johnston (1936) also propounded their theories on the marked differences in the growth of plants under different coloured light.

Seeing that it has been proven that coloured light, namely the visible rays, affects both plants and animals, surely it stands to reason that it must also affect man.

For many years, visible light has been used as a therapy on human beings, with some remarkable results. It has been shown that the visible rays work not only with the physical but also with the mental and spiritual aspects of man. In restoring these three aspects to harmony, a person becomes whole. One present-day researcher in this field is Theo Gimbel, who has shown how the visible rays do affect and help a person. To record but a few of his findings; he discovered that blue light reduces blood pressure, eases asthmatic attacks, helps insomnia and creates a state of relaxation and peace. At the opposite end of the spectrum, red has the reverse effect. It raises blood pressure and creates over-activity, but it is helpful in cases of anaemia. When he used orange light, he found that depression was lifted and replaced by a feeling of joy and happiness. He ascertained that green light dissolved virgin cell structure and was therefore very beneficial in cases of cancer. Turquoise he found helped to strengthen the immune system and reduce inflammation, therefore making it a very good colour for infections. Yellow helped arthritic sufferers by dissolving the calcium deposits in the joints.

Having myself been treated with colour and used it to treat others, and having also used it in conjunction with reflexology, I can only say that I have found it extremely beneficial and a powerful healer.

Knowing that science acknowledges that the electromagnetic waves at the top and bottom of the electromagnetic spectrum can affect human beings and uses these rays to treat illness, sometimes with horrendous side effects, why are scientists so unwilling to accept that the visible rays, which are the seven colours of the spectrum, can also affect a person and be used for healing with practically no side effects?

CHAPTER 2

The Subtle Anatomy

The Aura

The aura, which surrounds each person, is often referred to as an electromagnetic field. It is ovoid in shape, resembling an egg, the widest part being at the head and the narrowest part at the feet. Its width varies with each individual, depending upon their spiritual growth (see Figure 2 inside front cover).

The aura encompasses the emotions of a person in what is known as the astral body; the thoughts in what is called the mental body and past memories in what theosophists call the permanent atom. For a deeper insight into this subject I recommend *The Astral Body* and *The Mental Body* both written by A.E. Powell.

The aura is filled with energy patterns which determine the health of a person. Disease starts in the aura, caused by blockages in this energy flow. If these diseases are not cleared, then the disease manifests in the physical body.

The aura is filled with colours which are constantly changing according to our moods and well-being. The colours closest to the physical body are the densest, gradually becoming more ethereal as they move towards the outer edges of the aura. The luminosity of the colours again depends upon how advanced a soul is. In the aura of a young person, there appears a wide span of red around the lower part and a narrow span of magenta/white at the head. As a person matures, the abundance of red in the aura, the colour which earths a person to this planet, begins to diminish and is replaced by the expansion of the spiritual colours of magenta and white. When the time comes for the transition of the soul through death, the red colour is practically non-existent, the aura now being totally filled with magenta and white.

The aura is comprised of the auric bodies. These are the spiritual, causal, higher mental, mental, astral and etheric. These interpenetrate each other and the physical body.

The spiritual or bodyless body, as it is sometimes called, is the very essence of our being. It is the divine spark which is part of that ultimate reality or universal consciousness. It has no beginning and no ending.

The causal body contains the cause, the reason why we have reincarnated onto this planet. It contains the memory of all our previous lives, what we have learnt, what we still have to learn and the karma which we still have to work through. Karma is the law of cause and effect. As the master Christ said: 'Whatever ye sow so ye shall reap'.

The higher mental body is where inspirations and knowledge from the higher self manifest. These can then be absorbed into the lower mental body, if the channel between these two bodies has been opened. This is normally achieved through meditation and spiritual practices.

The lower mental body is filled with thought forms. Each thought that we and the rest of humanity thinks creates a form. If we think negative thoughts, they will attract other negative thoughts of a similar kind. Positive thoughts will attract positive thoughts. This is why it is important to change negative thinking into positive.

The astral body is our emotional body. In highly emotional people, this body is constantly fluctuating and therefore in a state of imbalance; a good reason why we should learn to control and resolve our emotions.

The body nearest to the physical body is the etheric or energy body. This contains the chakras and nadis, which are energy channels (Figure 3).

The Chakras and their Related Endocrine Glands

The word *chakra* is taken from the Sanskrit word meaning a wheel. These wheels are rotating energy centres within the body. They absorb *prana* or life force, break it up and distribute it through the nadis to the nervous system, the endocrine glands and the blood. There are seven major and twenty-one minor chakras. According to David Tansley in his book *Radionics and the Subtle Bodies of Man*, the seven major chakras are formed at points where the standing lines of light (lines of energy) cross each other twenty-one times. The twenty-one minor chakras are

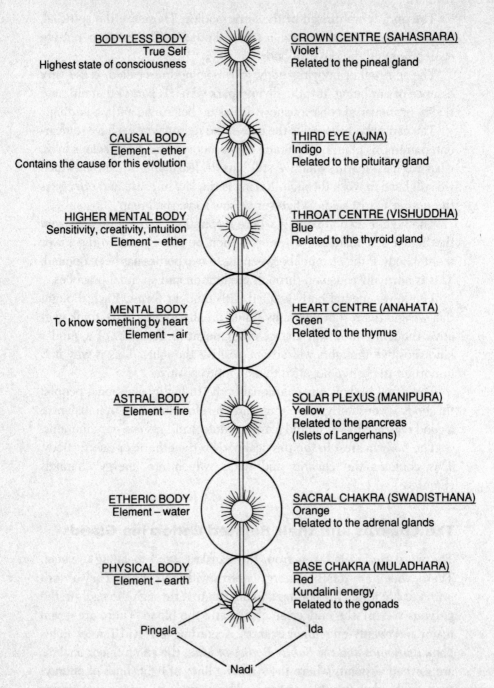

BODYLESS BODY
True Self
Highest state of consciousness

CROWN CENTRE (SAHASRARA)
Violet
Related to the pineal gland

CAUSAL BODY
Element – ether
Contains the cause for this evolution

THIRD EYE (AJNA)
Indigo
Related to the pituitary gland

HIGHER MENTAL BODY
Sensitivity, creativity, intuition
Element – ether

THROAT CENTRE (VISHUDDHA)
Blue
Related to the thyroid gland

MENTAL BODY
To know something by heart
Element – air

HEART CENTRE (ANAHATA)
Green
Related to the thymus

ASTRAL BODY
Element – fire

SOLAR PLEXUS (MANIPURA)
Yellow
Related to the pancreas
(Islets of Langerhans)

ETHERIC BODY
Element – water

SACRAL CHAKRA (SWADISTHANA)
Orange
Related to the adrenal glands

PHYSICAL BODY
Element – earth

BASE CHAKRA (MULADHARA)
Red
Kundalini energy
Related to the gonads

Pingala

Ida

Nadi

Fig. 3

located at points where the energy
strands cross fourteen times. Apart
from these, there are numerous
smaller chakras situated over the
body, where the energy lines cross
seven times. These points are used in
acupuncture.

The twenty-one minor chakras are
distributed thus: one in front of each
ear; one behind each eye; one on each
clavicle; one near the thymus gland;
one above each breast; one in the
palm of each hand (these being used
by contact healers); one near the liver;
one connected with the stomach; two
connected with the spleen; one related to each gonad; one behind each
knee and one on the sole of each foot
(Figure 4).

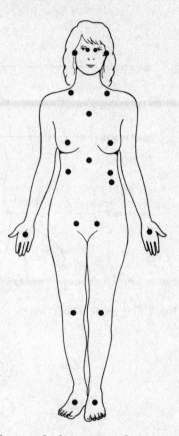

▷ **Fig. 4** The twenty-one minor chakras

The seven major chakras are situated in line with the spine. These are:
the crown centre which is just above the top of the head, the brow
chakra, the throat chakra, the heart chakra, the solar plexus chakra, the
sacral chakra and the base chakra. Each of these seven main chakras
works with one of the endocrine glands in the physical body. People
who are gifted with auric sight see these centres as discs of light. In a
young soul they are quite small, but as a person grows spiritually, so
they open into radiant saucers of light (Figures 5 and 6).

These chakras can become blocked or partially closed. This is
caused by trauma in a person's life. When this happens, the endocrine
glands are unable to function to their full potential and the physical
body suffers. It is therefore important to treat the chakras which are situated on the spinal reflex with both zone therapy and colour.

Each of these chakras contains all the colours of the spectrum, but
only one colour is dominant in each. Starting with the base centre and

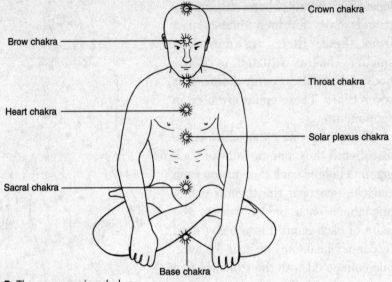

Fig. 5 The seven major chakras

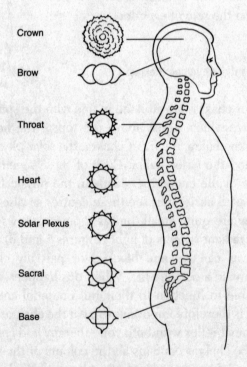

Fig. 6 The position of the chakras on the spine

working up to the crown, the dominant colours are red, orange, yellow, green, blue, indigo and violet.

Above the crown centre appear three higher chakras, about which very little is known. Information about these centres can be obtained through acknowledging their presence and working with them during meditation. The first of these radiates the colour magenta. The second, the pure white light of God-consciousness, and the third, the ultimate chakra, is black. This is the sacred black which contains all and out of which all things become manifest.

Realizing how important these energy centres are, let us look at them in more detail, with their associated glands.

The Muladhara or Base Chakra

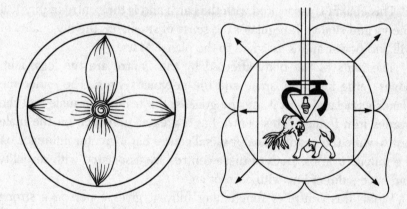

Muladhara translated means 'root' or 'base'. In eastern esoteric teaching it is symbolized by a deep red lotus flower with four petals. Barbara Ann Brennan, in her book *Hands of Light*, describes these petals as small rotating vortices which spin at a very high rate.

Inside the circle created by these petals is a yellow square, representing the earth and its stability. Radiating out from the square are six spears, projecting from the four corners and from the middle of the sides. These remind us of the many paths which are open to us as we travel along life's road. The animal associated with this chakra is an elephant with seven trunks. These are purported to signify the minerals needed to sustain physical life. Just above the elephant is a red triangle with its apex pointing downwards signifying the feminine aspect of creation. Within the triangle is a phallus or lingam around which is coiled a serpent. This is the kundalini, the serpent power. Above the phallus is a small crescent moon symbolizing the divine source of all energy. The deities which reside in this centre are Brahma and Dakini and the mantra or sound which it resonates to is LAM.

The muladhara is situated at the end of the coccyx and radiates downwards, thus connecting us to the earth. The colour of the rays which it emits is red, the colour which vibrates to the lowest frequency in the spectrum. This centre contains the primal energy, the kundalini shakti. It is said that when a person is ready mentally, physically and spiritually, the serpent will awaken and make her journey through each of the chakras to the crown chakra. Here she will bring enlightenment and realization.

This chakra is associated with the earth and is the centre of physical energy and vitality. It regulates the sense of smell, has the ray quality of will and power and is assigned to the planet Mars.

The parts of the body affected by this centre are the legs, feet, bones, large intestine, spine and the nervous system. The endocrine glands associated with it are the gonads; the testes in a male and the ovaries in a female. This centre has a greater influence on the male testes while the swadisthana or sacral centre has a greater influence on the female ovaries. Both of these centres are associated with sexuality and have a direct link with each other.

When this centre is functioning fully, it gives a person a strong will to live on the physical plane. He or she is filled with vitality and energy. Nothing is too much trouble and all of life becomes an exciting adventure.

If this centre is blocked, energy levels are low, making a person feel that they cannot be bothered to carry out their daily tasks. They have no enthusiasm for life.

The Gonads

The gonads are the male and female reproductive organs. In a male they are the testes and in a female the ovaries.

The ovaries, apart from producing ova, secrete the hormones oestrogen and progesterone. The secretion of oestrogen is influenced by the follicle stimulating hormone (FSH) which is produced by the pituitary gland. Oestrogen helps to regulate the menstrual cycle and develops the sexual characteristics of the female. Progesterone sensitizes the mucous membrane of the uterus in preparation for the fertilized ovum.

The male hormones produced by the testes are called androgens, and the most important is testosterone. This hormone is responsible for the changes which take place in a male during puberty.

The Swadisthana or Sacral Chakra

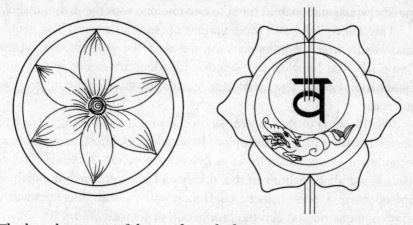

The literal meaning of the word *swadisthana* is 'one's own abode'. This chakra is situated halfway between the pubis and the navel, and is symbolized by an orange lotus with six petals which radiates the colour orange. Inside these petals is a crescent which houses an alligator. The white crescent symbolizes the moon, the symbol of female receptivity. It is associated with the water element and affects the flow of fluids in the body. The presiding deities are Vishnu and Rakini and the mantra or sound is VAM.

This centre is ruled by the moon and has love and wisdom as its ray qualities. The energy radiated here is of a much finer quality than the 'down to earth' energy of the base centre.

This centre is associated with sex and does not awaken until puberty. The sexual energy is the second most powerful energy in a human being, the first being the life force of the base centre. This centre has an affinity with the fifth or throat centre and in certain tantric practices and disciplines, the sexual energy from this centre can be transmuted to the throat centre where it is used for creativity and communication. This creativity also applies to the higher worlds. Sexual alchemy uses this centre for personal transformation but this needs strict physical and mental control.

Practitioners of tantric yoga can use this sexual energy in two ways. Firstly, with a partner, they use sexual union as a way of uniting themselves with the cosmic consciousness. The second way is by transmuting this energy within themselves in order to unite the feminine and masculine energies resident in themselves. This uniting is said to make a person whole and enables them to become one with the divine reality.

This centre links with the emotions of fear and anxiety. The glands and organs which it influences are the skin, the reproductive organs (especially the female), the kidneys, bladder, circulatory system and lymphatic system. The endocrine glands associated with it are the adrenals.

The blocking of this centre may result in a woman being unable to reach orgasm during sexual union. In a male it manifests as premature ejaculation or the inability to achieve an erection. Other disorders caused are abnormalities in the kidney and bladder functions such as infections and poor urinary control, problems with the circulatory system, menstruation and the production of seminal fluids.

When this centre is functioning to its full potential, it opens the intuitive and psychic powers. When it first awakens, it can upset the sexual energies and heighten awareness to external stimuli. These will again find their own balance but on a higher level of consciousness.

The Adrenal Glands

There are two adrenal glands, one situated on the top of each kidney. They are about 1 inch in length and yellowish in colour. They contain an outer cortex and an interior or medulla.

The cortex is responsible for secreting substances known as steroids. These are divided into three main groups.

Group A These are the mineral corticoids. They work on the tubules of the kidneys to help retain sodium and chloride in the body and to aid in the excretion of excess potassium.

Group B   These are the gluco-corticoids. These assist in the conversion of carbohydrates into glycogen. They increase the blood sugar, help in the utilization of fat, decrease the number of lymphocytes and eosinophils in the blood and reduce the rate at which certain connective tissue cells multiply. This action tends to suppress the natural reaction to healing and therefore delays it. The other hormones in this group are cortisone and hydrocortisone.

Group C   These are similar to the hormones produced by the gonads. They influence growth and sex development in males and females.

The hormones secreted by the cortex are influenced by the adrenocorticotrophic hormone (ACTH), secreted by the pituitary gland.

The medulla of the adrenal glands secretes adrenaline and noradrenaline. Adrenaline stimulates the sympathetic nervous system and causes the arteries of the body to constrict. This results in an increase in the heart beat and a rise in blood pressure. Adrenaline also stimulates the liver into converting glycogen into glucose, which is used during muscle activity. The adrenals are often called the 'fight or flight glands' because they pour adrenaline into the blood in times of stress, danger or excitement in order to stimulate the body into action.

Addison's Disease   This is caused by the adrenal glands becoming diseased in adult life. The symptoms are low blood pressure, digestive disturbances and a brown pigmentation of the skin and mucous membranes.

Cushing's Syndrome   This is caused by the over-secretion of hydrocortisone. It produces rounding of the face (moon face), obesity, hypertension, diabetes and osteoporosis.

The Manipura or Solar Plexus Chakra

The word *manipura* means 'city of jewels' or 'filled with jewels'. This centre is so called because it is the fire centre, the focal point of heat which radiates like a golden sun.

In Chinese philosophy it is called the triple warmer because during the process of digestion, heat is generated. In Japanese teaching it is called the *Hara* which translated means 'belly'. Many esoteric schools teach overtone singing to activate the energies of this centre.

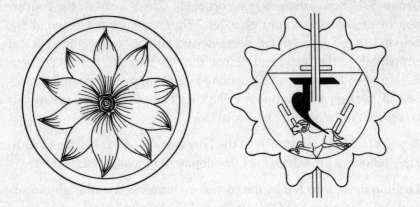

It is situated between the twelfth thoracic and the first lumbar vertebrae. It is depicted as a bright yellow lotus with ten petals. In the centre is a downward-pointing red triangle with a T-shaped projection on each of its three sides. The animal of this chakra is the ram and the mantra or sound is RAM. The deities are Rudra, the god of storms, and Lakini, the goddess of good fortune.

This is the centre of vitality in the psychic and physical bodies because it is the centre where *prana* (the upward-moving vitality) and *apana* (the downward-moving vitality) meet, generating the heat that is necessary to support life. When these two energies are joined, this centre is awakened. It is ruled by the sun and has the ray quality of active intelligence.

On the astral or emotional level, this centre is connected to desire and the emotions. It is involved in people who lack confidence and courage.

On the physical level, this centre is chiefly concerned with the process of digestion and absorption. The glands, processes and organs influenced by this chakra are the breath, the diaphragm, stomach, duodenum, gall bladder and liver. The endocrine gland associated with it is the pancreas.

When this chakra is unstable, a person can be subjected to rapid mood swings and may suffer from depression, introversion, lethargy, poor digestion and abnormal eating habits. Its malfunction can lead to nervous instability and to cancer, if the energies from the heart centre fail to be expressed on the physical plane. This centre interacts between the heart and sacral centre and if it is blocked, then sexuality cannot be connected to love. When this centre is open, a deep and fulfilling emotional life is experienced.

This centre is also related to inner connectedness. When two people enter into a friendship, cords are formed between their solar plexuses. The stronger the relationship, the stronger the cords. If the relationship ends, the cords are slowly disconnected. A similar cord is formed between a mother and her newborn child.

The Pancreas

The pancreas is situated behind the stomach and lies transversely across the posterior abdominal wall at the level of the first and second lumbar vertebrae. It is a gland similar in structure to the salivary glands. It has an external and an internal secretion. The external secretion is insulin.

Only part of the pancreas is endocrine. These are the islets of Langerhans which secrete the insulin responsible for the metabolism of sugar. Without insulin, the muscles are unable to use the sugar, which circulates in the blood, for energy. Sugar is used by the tissues in the form of glucose. In order to produce energy, this is broken down into carbon dioxide and water. Any excess of sugar in the blood is stored in the liver as glycogen. If the blood sugar is too high, the excess is excreted by the kidneys and appears in the urine.

If the islets of Langerhans do not function properly, due to disease, there is a lack of insulin and this results in diabetes. This is a condition where the blood sugar is too high. It is normally diagnosed through the appearance of sugar in the urine.

The Anahata or Heart Chakra

The word *anahata* means the 'unstruck'. All sound in the universe is produced by striking objects together. This sets up vibrations or sound waves. The primordial sound, which comes from beyond this world, is the source of all sound and is known as the anahata sound. This centre is where the sound manifests. It is also at this centre that the path towards higher consciousness starts.

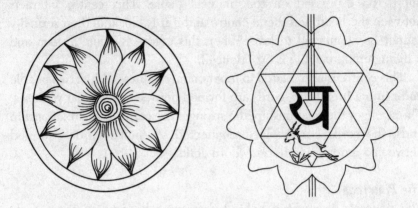

This chakra is situated between the fourth and fifth thoracic vertebrae and is symbolized by a green lotus with twelve petals. In the centre of the lotus is a hexagram (as in the Star of David). It is associated with the element of air and the sense of touch. Its ruling planet is Venus and its ray quality is harmony through conflict. The mantra which vibrates with this centre is YAM. The animal depicted is an antelope and the deities are Isha and Kakini.

On the physical level, anahata is associated with the heart and circulatory system, the lungs and respiratory system, the immune system and the arms and hands. The endocrine gland that it is attributed to is the thymus.

This is the centre through which we love. Love can be expressed on many levels. It can be purely selfish, demanding and constricting or it can be compassionate and caring. The more open this centre is, the greater our capacity to extend undemanding spiritual love. It is through this centre that we connect with those with whom we have a love relationship. When this centre is open, we can perceive the beauty and spiritual love in our fellow human beings. Its awakening brings a greater sensitivity to touch and a detachment from material objects.

Situated just below the heart chakra is a smaller centre which is represented by a red lotus with eight petals. This chakra is known as the *kalparvriksha* or kalpa tree. Inside this lotus is depicted an island of gems. It contains a jewelled altar where a devotee may come in meditation to meet his guru. The following description of this centre is taken from *Yoga* by Ernest Wood.

Let him find in his heart a broad ocean of nectar,
Within it a beautiful island of gems,
Where the sands are bright golden and sprinkled with jewels,
Fair trees line its shores with a myriad of blooms,
And within it rare bushes, trees, creepers and rushes,
On all sides shed fragrance most sweet to the sense.

Who would taste of the sweetness of divine completeness
Should picture therein a most wonderful tree,
On whose far spreading branches grow fruit of all fancies,
The four mighty teachings that hold up the world.
There the fruit and the flowers know no death and no sorrows,
While to them the bees hum and soft cuckoos sing.

Now, under the shadow of that peaceful arbour
A temple of rubies most radiant is seen.
And he who shall seek there will find on a seat rare,
His dearly beloved enshrined therein.
Let him dwell with his mind, as his teacher defines
On that Divine Form, with its modes and its signs.

The Thymus Gland

This gland is situated in the thorax, behind the sternum and in front of the heart. It mainly consists of lymphoid tissue and plays a part in the formation of lymphocytes. At birth, this gland is quite large and continues to increase in size until puberty when it then starts to get smaller. The thymus plays an important part in the body's immune system.

It is claimed that certain yogic practices can keep this gland active, thereby keeping a person youthful and the immune system strong.

The Vishuddha or Throat Chakra

The word *vishuddha* means to purify, hence this chakra is the centre of purification. It is symbolized by a smoky violet blue lotus with sixteen petals. In the centre of the lotus is a downward-pointing triangle containing a white circle. This chakra is associated with the element of ether and the sense of hearing. It is connected with the planet Mercury and its ray quality is concrete science and knowledge. The animal depicted is an elephant, the deities are Sadasiva and Sakini, and the mantra or sound is HAM.

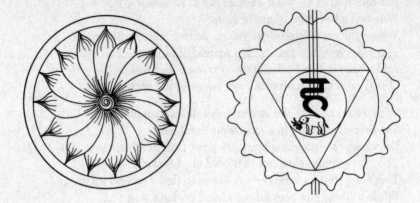

The throat centre is reported to be the place where divine nectar (the mystical elixir of immortality) is tasted. This nectar is a kind of sweet secretion produced by the gland known as the *lalana chakra* which is located near the back of the throat. The nectar gland is stimulated by higher yogic practices and the nectar can sustain a yogi for any length of time without food or water.

On the physical level, this chakra governs the nervous system, female reproductive organs, the vocal chords and the ears. The endocrine glands associated with it are the thyroid and parathyroids.

The throat chakra is the creative centre, especially of the spoken word. The use of this centre in communication is unique to humanity. In Tibetan mysticism, each sound is valued as a vibration, an invisible energy, and therefore only uttered when necessary. Today we talk end-lessly about nothing in particular and through this, our sense of sound has become deadened. In eastern esotericism, sound has always been used in the form of mantras to heighten the awareness and level of con-sciousness. This was introduced in the west by the Maharishi Mahesh Yogi in the form of TM (transcendental meditation).

This centre is used for singing. Music produced by the voice is very therapeutic. Medieval Christian monastic infirmaries used music to help people in pain, to comfort the terminally ill and support a conscious death. Contemplative musicians in Denver, USA, have re-established this tradition. Eighteen years ago, Therese Schroeder-Sheker formed a group called the Chalice midwives who employ harp and voice in assisting the entire process of death and dying in home, hospital and hospice. Their work with pain resolution and the possibility of a conscious death is particularly attentive to the restoration of dignity, intimacy and reverence within the personal and community experience of death. This is described in her book *The Luminous Wound*.

The throat centre is the bridge which one crosses from the physical into the spiritual realm. When this chakra is open, communication with old friends can become awkward, as entering into the spiritual realm changes one's energies and former friends, feeling these changes, find it difficult to communicate with the spiritual energies. But these new energies start to attract new friends of a like mind. As this centre awakens, it brings with it the gift of telepathy and the knowledge of past, present and future.

Imbalances in this centre can lead to asthma, vertigo, allergies, anaemia, fatigue, laryngitis, sore throats and menstrual problems. It can also cause a tendency towards skin and respiratory problems. Feelings of emptiness and difficulties with self-expression may also be experienced.

The Thyroid Gland
The thyroid gland is situated in the lower part of the neck. It consists of two lobes, which are situated on either side of the trachea and joined together by an isthmus which passes in front of the trachea. The active hormones of this gland are thyroxine and triodothyronine. These contain a high percentage of iodine. One of the main functions of the thyroid gland is to restore iodine in the body. The secretion of thyroxine is regulated by the thyroid stimulating hormone (TSH) which is secreted by the anterior lobe of the pituitary gland.

The functions of this gland are:

a) controlling the metabolism of the body;
b) keeping the skin and hair in good condition;
c) affecting the irritability of the nervous system;
d) co-operating with the other ductless glands to keep the endocrine balance in the body;
e) controlling the body growth and mental development in infancy;
f) storing iodine.

Over-secretion of the hormones produces a disease called thyrotoxicosis. This is generally associated with a goitre which is an enlargement of the thyroid gland. The symptoms are protrusion of the eyeballs, rapid pulse, increased sweating and general nervousness. Even though a person eats well, they are normally thin due to the increased metabolic rate. Because of the effect of this over-secretion on the other ductless glands, disturbances occur in the menstrual cycle.

Under-secretion of this gland differs in adults and children. In adults, it is known as myxoedema, and the symptoms are the reverse of those in over-secretion. The person tends to gain in weight, the skin is dry and thick and the hair scanty. The metabolic rate is slowed down, causing difficulty in keeping warm. In infancy the condition is known as cretinism and causes stunted growth and failure of mental development.

The Parathyroid Glands

There are four parathyroid glands, each one about the size of a pea, and situated behind each of the four poles of the thyroid gland. The hormone they secrete is parathormone which controls the calcium metabolism of the body. Under-secretion of this hormone gives rise to a condition known as tetany. With this condition the body is unable to mobilize and use calcium, thus the calcium content of the blood is low. Symptoms are muscular spasms and increased irritability of the nervous system. Over-secretion gives rise to an increase of calcium in the blood and urine and leads to osteitis fibrosa which is a disease of the bone.

The Ajna or Brow Chakra

The word ajna means 'command' and it is at this centre that one receives commands from the higher self. It is depicted as having two petals and is situated at the centre of the brow. This centre is sometimes referred to as the third eye and when awakened it acts as a third eye with the development of the gifts of telepathy and knowing.

The chakra is symbolized by a circle containing a golden downward-pointing triangle. Its mantra is OM and the deities are Sakti Hakini and Shiva. It is ruled by the planet Uranus and has devotion and idealism as its ray qualities.

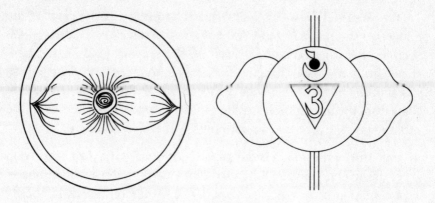

The two petals represent the ego self and the spirit self; the reasoning and the intuitive mind. At this centre the two main nadis, the *ida* (masculine) and the *pingala* (feminine), meet and the feminine and masculine aspects of a person merge, bringing about a spiritual awakening.

Ajna is frequently used as a centre for concentration during meditation. Through its awakening, one develops the gifts of clairvoyance, clairaudience and telepathy. It is sometimes referred to as the door which leads to deeper and higher realms of awareness. Through this chakra a person can increase the powers of intelligence, memory, willpower, concentration and visualization. When this centre is fully awakened, we are beyond our own karma (having reached the level on our spiritual path where the law of cause and effect is no longer relevant to us) but are able to see the karma of those around us and of nations of the world. When we are centred in this chakra, we are given the power to help others to dissolve their karma.

On the physical level, it is related to the eyes, nose, ears and brain. Instability in this centre leads to tiredness, irritability, confusion and rigid thoughts.

Imbalances can lead to sinus problems, catarrh, hay fever, sleeplessness, mental stress, neuritis and migraine. The endocrine gland with which it is associated is the pituitary.

The Pituitary Gland

The pituitary gland is about 1 cm in diameter and is situated at the base of the brain. It consists of an anterior and posterior lobe, both having different modes of development and entirely different functions.

The anterior lobe is frequently referred to as the master gland of the endocrine system. It is under the influence of the hypothalamus which secretes releasing factors for each of the trophic hormones. These travel from the hypothalamus to the anterior pituitary gland in the blood of the portal system which runs in the pituitary stalk. The secretions from the anterior lobe of the pituitary control the activities of the other endocrine glands. The hormones which it secretes are:

a) somatrotrophin which is the growth hormone (GH). Over-secretion of this in childhood leads to excessive growth in the length of bones, a condition known as gigantism. Under-secretion results in obesity and disorders of carbohydrate metabolism. Sexual development may also be defective;
b) the thyroid stimulating hormone (TSH);
c) the adrenocorticotrophic hormone (ACTH). This hormone is a protein substance which stimulates the cortex of the adrenal glands to secrete its own hormones;
d) the gonadotrophic hormones (GTH). These are essential for the normal development of sex organs and stimulate the production of the various sex gland hormones;
e) prolactin. This is the lactogenic hormone which helps to control the secretion of milk from the breast.

The posterior lobe secretes two hormones: vasopressin and oxytocin. Vasopressin is an antidiuretic hormone (ADH) which concentrates the urine by increasing the absorption of water in the distal renal tubules. It raises blood pressure and causes contraction of involuntary muscles, especially of the intestines and bladder. Oxytocin stimulates the muscles of the uterus during and immediately after labour. It also stimulates the lactating breast to secrete milk.

The Sahasrara or Crown Chakra

The *sahasrara* chakra is situated just above the crown of the head. It is symbolized as a thousand-petalled lotus, which represents infinity. This chakra leads us into the eternal, infinite, supreme existence. It is the centre of pure consciousness and the abode of Shiva. When the kundalini rises, Shiva and Shakti are united, bringing about a

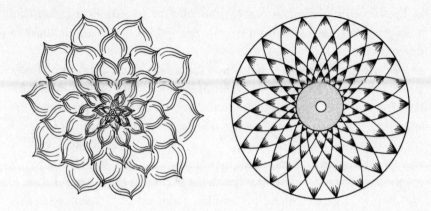

transformation in human consciousness. (In Hinduism, Shakti is the Goddess principle or power. Shiva is the aspect of Divine power which is responsible for raising man from physical bondage to spiritual enlightenment. Through the higher practices of yoga, in conjunction with meditation upon the chakras, the earth power (Shakti) travels through the chakras to become harmonized with the spiritual power of Shiva.) When we have reached this state we have attained realization and transcended the need to reincarnate into a physical body, unless we choose to do so in order to help humanity. This centre is ruled by the planet Neptune and has the ray quality of ceremonial white magic. There is no mantra for the crown chakra.

Sahasrara is situated outside the physical body and is mainly connected with the higher consciousness of the true self. The colour violet which radiates from it is the colour of dignity, self-respect and healing. The endocrine gland associated with it is the pineal.

When this centre is open, a person sees his or her spirituality in a very personal way; a spirituality that is not tied up with any dogma. The full awakening of this centre enables a person to work with the three higher chakras mentioned on page 13.

The Pineal Gland

The pineal gland is a small reddish-grey structure about the size of a pea. It is situated between the under-surface of the cerebrum and the mid-brain, just in front of the cerebellum. Its main secretion is melatonin which affects the body's biological clock. The level of melatonin in the blood is highest at night, gradually decreasing during the day. This gland regulates the onset of puberty, induces sleep and influences our moods.

We are light beings which have incarnated into a physical body. Jacob Liberman, in his book *Light: Medicine of the Future*, reiterates this. He states that natural light containing the ultraviolet portion of the spectrum is vital to our well-being. He says that light entering the eyes is not only used to aid our vision but activates our biological clock by way of the pineal gland and hypothalamus. The hypothalamus is responsible for controlling the functions that keep the body in balance.

I believe that this gland is stimulated during meditation, secreting hormones which can take us into those higher states of consciousness. It can produce the same experiences as those provoked by LSD, but far more safely. This gland is sometimes referred to as the hallucinatory gland. Yoga philosophy teaches that it is the link between the gross physical body and the more subtle psychic body.

The Splenic Chakra

The splenic chakra is not a major chakra but is of great importance. It has six petals or spokes and is found where two minor centres join over the spleen. This is the centre where prana is absorbed.

Prana is the life force which exists in animals, plants and humans, and in humans it manifests on the physical, astral and mental levels. Its manifestation on the physical plane appears to depend upon sunlight. Prana emanates from the sun and enters some of the physical atoms which float about in the earth's atmosphere in countless numbers, and causes them to glow. On a sunny day prana is in abundance, on a cloudy day it is greatly reduced and at night it is practically non-existent. It seems that at night we use the prana which has been manufactured during the previous day. At night, when the body is asleep, the nerves and muscles relax and the assimilation of prana takes place. This is the reason for the strong recuperative power of sleep, even if it be just a short nap.

The splenic chakra absorbs the vitality globules from the atmosphere and breaks them up into the seven variations of prana, each radiating its own colour. The remaining seven chakras absorb and distribute this prana to the etheric and then to the physical body. The seven varieties of prana radiate rose red, dark red, orange, yellow, green, blue and violet. The indigo of the spectrum is divided between the violet and blue rays, whilst the red is split up into dark red and rose red prana. Each of the six petals or spokes of this chakra takes one of the different kinds of prana and distributes it to the part of the body to which it is affiliated. The seventh variety, which is rose pink, passes through the centre of the chakra and is distributed over the whole of the nervous system. If a person lacks this colour he or she may be sensitive, intensely irritable, restless and the least noise or touch is extremely painful. This can be alleviated by flooding the person with rose pink.

The Spleen

The spleen is situated behind the lower ribs on the left side of the abdomen.

The spleen is not an endocrine gland and is not known to produce any important internal secretion. It is better described as a lymphatic organ as most of this gland is made up of lymphoid tissue and is surrounded by a fibrous capsule.

The main functions of the spleen are the destruction of old, worn-out red blood corpuscles, the production of some antibodies and the defence of the body against infection, the provision of some of the lymphocytes in the blood, and sometimes the destruction of platelets.

From a medical point of view, the spleen is not essential to life and can be removed without any permanent damage to health.

CHAPTER 3

The Structure of the Feet

Reflexologists are working most of the time with patients' feet. I therefore feel that it is important to know their anatomy so that we can correctly and more easily locate the reflexes.

Each foot contains twenty-six bones and thirty-three articulations which are joined together by over 100 ligaments. The twenty-six bones are:

The calcaneus
The talus
The navicular
The cuboid
3 cuneiform bones
5 metatarsals
14 phalanges (the big toe contains two phalanges and the remaining four toes contain three each) (see Figure 7)

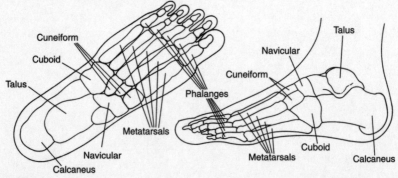

Fig. 7 Bone structure of the foot

The talus and calcaneus are situated on the posterior part of the foot. The anterior part of the foot contains the cuboid, navicular and three cuneiform bones. The word *cuneiform* means 'wedge-shaped'; these three bones are referred to as the medial, intermediate and lateral cuneiform. The talus is the only bone in the foot that articulates with the fibula and tibia bones of the leg. When one is walking, the talus initially bears the entire weight of the body. Part of this weight is then transmitted to the calcaneus and the remainder to the other tarsal bones. The heel bone or calcaneus is the largest and strongest bone in the foot.

There are five metatarsal bones, each one comprising a proximal base and a shaft with a distal head. These bones articulate proximally with the first, second and third cuneiform bones and with the cuboid; distally, they articulate with the phalanges. The first metatarsal is thicker than the rest and bears more weight.

Like the metatarsal bones, the phalanges also consist of a proximal base, a middle shaft and a distal head. The hallux or big toe has two large, heavy phalanges known as the proximal and distal phalanges. The other four toes each consist of three phalanges. If a person wears tightly fitting shoes, the big toe can become deformed into what is commonly known as a bunion. This condition can be inherited. Another problem which can occur is arthritis of the first metatarsophalangeal joint. This produces inflammation of the fluid-filled sacs (bursae) at the joint, bone spurs and calluses.

The bones of the feet are arranged in such a way that they form two arches, the longitudinal and the transverse arch (Figure 8). The longitudinal arch consists of the medial or inner part and the lateral or outer part. These arches enable the foot to support the weight of the body and provide leverage while walking. The bones which make up these arches are held in position by tendons and ligaments. If these tendons and ligaments are weakened, the height of the medial longitudinal arch may decrease or fall. This results in a condition known as flatfoot. If the medial longitudinal arch is abnormally elevated, frequently caused by a muscle imbalance, a condition known as clawfoot occurs.

The muscles of the foot are intricate and are comparable to those of the hand but, whereas the muscles in the hand are specialized for precise and intricate movements, those of the foot are limited to support and locomotion. The muscles of the foot are divided into two groups, the dorsal and plantar. There is only one dorsal muscle and this is the extensor digitorum brevis. The plantar muscles are arranged in four layers. The first layer consists of the abductor hallucis, flexor digitorum brevis and the abductor digiti minimi. The second layer comprises the quadratus plantae and the lumbricals. The third layer is the flexor hallucis brevis, adductor hallucis and the flexor digiti minimi brevis. The fourth layer consists of the dorsal interossei and the plantar interossei.

All of these muscles are responsible for the movement of the toes and the foot.

Comfortable and properly functioning feet are essential for the well-being of the whole body. Painful, abnormal feet can lead to bad posture, fatigue, muscular cramp and backache.

The feet support the weight of the body and act as levers to raise the body and move it forward. It is therefore important that one's feet should be kept in good condition. The nails should be kept short and hard skin removed. It has been shown that if the nail of the big toe is too long and presses into the side of the toe (part of the head reflex), headaches can occur. Many people's feet have been deformed by wearing ill-fitting shoes. This is detrimental to health because the reflexes which occur at the site of the deformity are affected. Ideally we should walk barefooted whenever possible, allowing the feet to move freely and the skin to breathe.

Before carrying out a reflexology treatment, visual observation of the feet should be made. The things to look for are any abnormalities in the bone structure, colour of the skin and temperature of the feet. These could give an indication that there is disease in the body. For

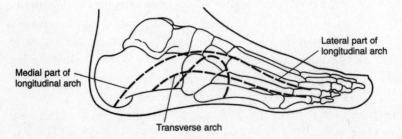

Fig. 8 The arches of the foot

example, an alteration in the tonus of the skin beneath the phalanges of the second and third toes could indicate eye problems; hard skin, corns or calluses over a reflex could reveal a problem in the corresponding part of the physical body. The more you practise this visual art, the more you will come to realize how much information can be gleaned about a person through the condition of their feet.

CHAPTER 4

Reflexology

A Short History

Reflexology was rediscovered by Dr William Fitzgerald, who was born in Middletown, USA, in 1872. In 1895 he graduated in medicine at the University of Vermont, and then practised at hospitals in Vienna, Paris and London before specializing in ear, nose and throat disorders. He died in Stamford, USA, in 1942.

Early this century, he began to consider the possibility of treating the body through pressure points found on the feet. In his book on zone therapy he says:

> A form of treatment by means of pressure points was known in India and China 5,000 years ago. This knowledge, however, appears to be lost or forgotten. Perhaps it was set aside in favour of acupuncture which emerged as the stronger growth from the same root.

If we look back in history, we can find evidence of this technique being used. Cellini (1500–1571), the great Florentine sculptor, is reported to have used strong pressure on his fingers and toes in order to relieve pain in his body, with great success. Likewise, W. Garfield (1831–81), an American president, is supposed to have alleviated the pain of an assassination attempt by applying pressure to various points on his feet. Apparently, all other medication prescribed had failed.

North American Indian tribes knew the relationship between the reflex points and the internal organs of the body and used this knowledge to treat disease. It is still used in Indian reservations.

In 1916, a Dr E. Bowers publicly described the treatment propounded by Dr Fitzgerald and called it 'Zone Therapy'. In 1917, their combined work appeared in a book called *Zone Therapy*. It contained therapeutic proposals and recommendations for doctors, dentists, gynaecologists, ear, nose and throat specialists, and chiropractors. Diagrams of the reflexes of the feet and the corresponding division of the ten zones of the body appeared in the first edition of this book, and Dr Fitzgerald started to teach this method of treatment to practitioners by giving courses of instruction.

An American masseuse, Eunice Ingham, became interested in this method and started to learn more about it. She spent many years gaining insight into how it worked and developed a special subtle method of massage called the Ingham method of compression massage. This is described in her book *Stories the Feet Can Tell*. Reflexology is thought to have been brought to England by Doreen Bayley who was a pupil of Eunice Ingham.

According to the medical dictionary, the word 'reflex' means an involuntary muscle contraction due to an external stimulus and relayed by a central organ such as the spinal cord. In the context of reflex zone therapy, the word 'reflex' is not used in this sense but in the sense of reflecting the entire organism, head, neck and trunk, on a small screen which is the feet.

Reflexology teaches that a vital energy called life force or prana circulates in a balanced rhythmic way between all the organs of the body. It also permeates every living cell and tissue. If this energy becomes blocked, the organ relating to the blockage becomes dis-eased. Also, bacteria and virus-related diseases can upset the energy balance in the body.

The human system, functioning in accordance with the law of polarity, has two main points. One of these is at the top of the head and the other at the feet. Between these two poles, ten separate energy currents circulate, five in each half of the body, between the head and the toes and the five fingers. These currents flow in perpendicular lines called zones and within these zones lie all the organs and muscles of the body (Figures 9 and 10).

Apart from these energy zones, the feet are further divided into three transverse zones. The first division lies between the phalanges and metatarsals; above this, in zone 1, are the reflexes to the head and neck. The second division lies between the metatarsals, the cuneiform and cuboid bones. Above this in zone 2 are found the reflexes to the chest and upper abdomen. The third division lies midway between the calcaneus and the talus bone. Above it are the reflexes to the abdomen and pelvis. Learning the positions of these zones on the feet makes it much easier to locate the exact position of the reflexes (Figure 11).

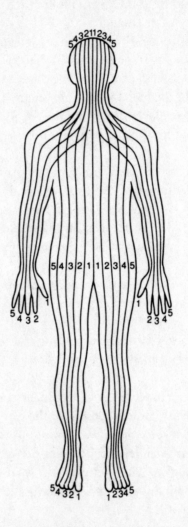

Fig. 9 The ten energy zones of the body

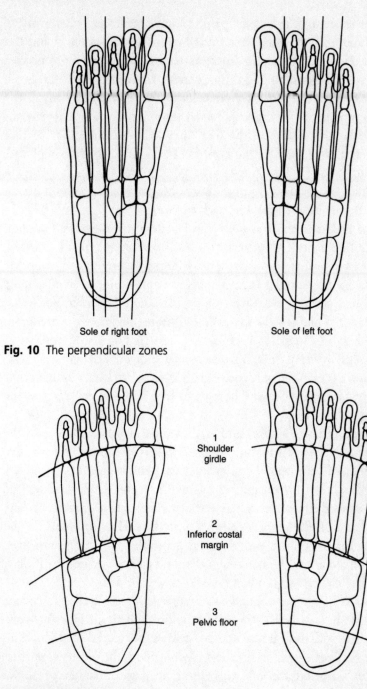

Sole of right foot   Sole of left foot

Fig. 10 The perpendicular zones

1
Shoulder
girdle

2
Inferior costal
margin

3
Pelvic floor

Fig. 11 The transverse zones

The soles of our feet and the palms of our hands are a mirror image of the whole body because it is here that energy terminates and the reflexes are found. The energy terminating on the feet is more powerful than that terminating on the hands, therefore it is far more beneficial to treat the feet. If there is an energy blockage in any of the zones, then pain will be experienced by the patient when that particular area is being treated on the feet. It is to these painful areas that colour is administered after the normal treatment has been completed. The correct colour will help to release the blockage and allow the life force to flow freely again. Another advantage of using colour is that these blockages can be released without pain.

Energy blocks in the zones can have many causes. Stress, bad diet, a life style that is no longer correct, a broken marriage or relationship, to name but a few. If the dis-ease is going to be eradicated, then the cause has to be found. This can take many hours of counselling. Sometimes a person can bury it deep in their subconscious mind because it is too painful to cope with. Other people know the cause but are unwilling to discuss it because they are not ready to resolve it. These blocks are frequently hurdles over which we must go if we wish to grow and evolve, but only too often it is easier to stay where we are. This is our choice. We have been given free will and nobody has the right to take this away.

The importance of finding and eradicating the cause is shown by the patient who came with chronic sinusitis. During counselling, we discussed diet and he revealed that he ate vast quantities of dairy produce. This is well known for producing mucus in the body. He was advised that if he wished to be free of his condition he should eliminate all dairy produce from his diet, and he agreed to do this. He continued regular treatment but very little progress was achieved. He was again questioned on his diet and he confessed that he had tried to come off dairy produce but as yet had not had the will-power to do so.

I heard a lovely story about a lady who was terminally ill with cancer. Her one wish was to see the world before she died. Her husband, knowing this, sold their house and possessions so that he could fulfil his wife's wish. They went on a cruise, seeing many beautiful countries. When they returned, the wife was cured, no trace of cancer left in her body. Obviously, the complete change was what she needed.

If the cause cannot be found, then a patient will continue to block the energy which the reflexologist has released. Equally, as shown by the first example, if the cause is known and the patient has no wish or desire to work with it, then the energy channels which the reflexologist frees will be blocked again by the patient. Unlike conventional medicine where a patient is given a prescription and has to take no responsibility for him or herself, in complementary medicine the opposite applies. A patient is expected to take responsibility and work with him or herself and the therapist to effect a cure.

The Reflexes of the Feet

Assuming that people reading this book are already qualified reflexologists or are training to become one and are reading this book because they are interested in using colour with their treatment, I do not intend to go into great detail about the reflexes of the hands and feet and the methods of treatment. This has already been covered in the many excellent books available on the market and I feel that to repeat what has already been written serves no purpose. What I do feel is that, when one is giving a reflexology treatment, it is important to work to a set order. This ensures that none of the reflexes is inadvertently omitted. It is also important to know the exact position of the pressure points and for this purpose I have included the bone structure in the diagrams of the reflex zones found on the feet (Figures 12–16).

Before the first patient of the day arrives, I always light a candle asking that I may be a channel through which the healing power of the universe flows. This candle can represent the Christ light, the Buddha light or the pure universal light. It is important to remember that none of us are healers, but our physical body, the temple in which we live, when sensitized and open can become a most beautiful instrument and channel through which the healing energy flows.

When giving a reflexology treatment, it should not be carried out as a purely mechanical therapy. During the time of treatment, the auras of the patient and the therapist come into contact. If therapists are sensitive to this, they should be able to feel into the patient and to detect problems and blockages which the patient feels unable to talk about. This knowledge can help a great deal when one is trying to bring a

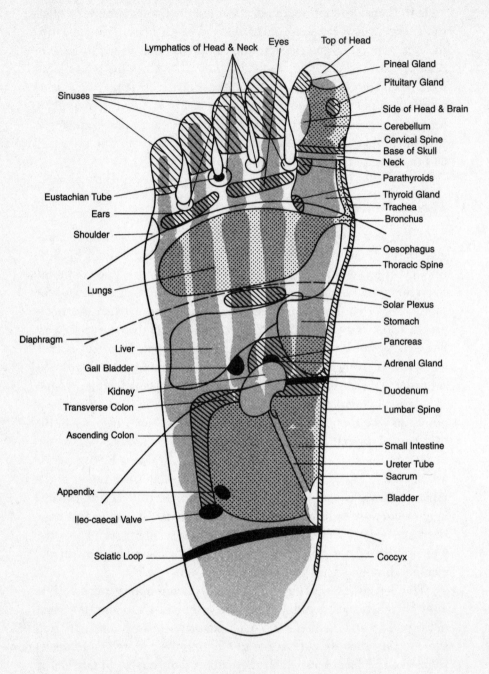

Fig. 12 Reflexes of the right foot as viewed from underneath

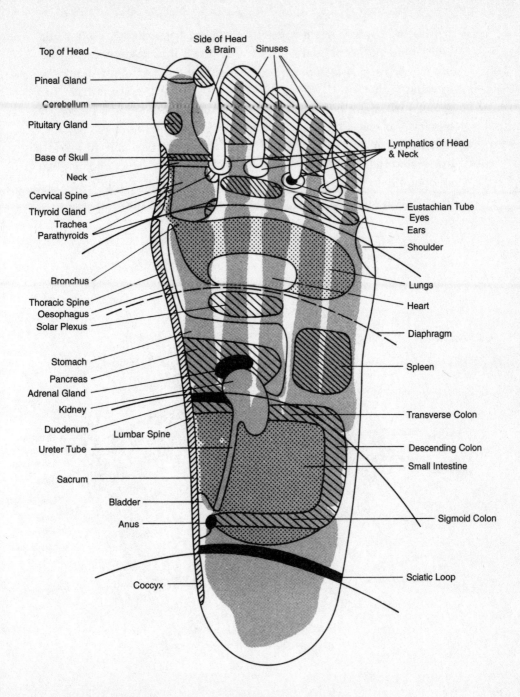

Fig. 13 Reflexes of the left foot as viewed from underneath

person back into harmony. Each of us is a triple being, comprising body, mind and spirit, and it is only when these three aspects are in harmony that we can become whole. Therefore, all treatment should be working with these three levels of being. Some therapists have the gift of auric sight; being able to see the aura surrounding a person. If one has this gift, I feel that it should not be used without the patient's permission. A person's aura reveals, to those who are able to read it, everything that there is to know about that person. They become like an open book. To be able to work constructively with this gift, one has to learn to 'switch it on and off' and to use it responsibly.

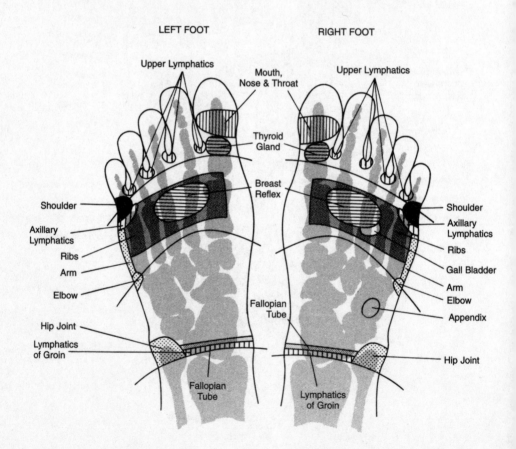

Fig. 14 Reflexes on top of the foot

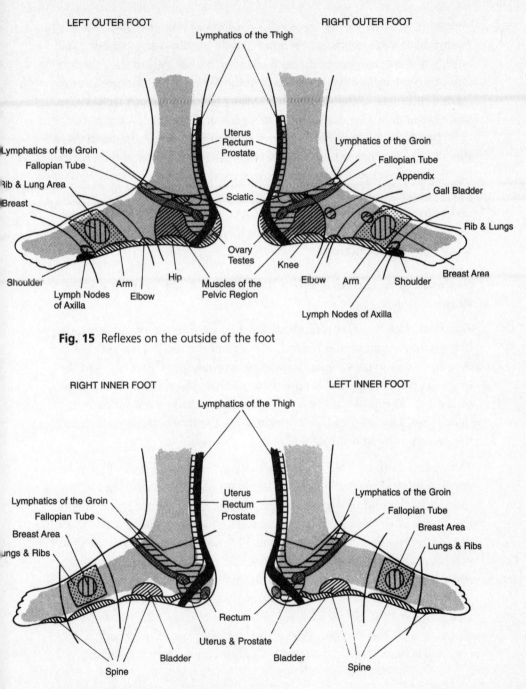

LEFT OUTER FOOT

RIGHT OUTER FOOT

Lymphatics of the Thigh

Lymphatics of the Groin

Fallopian Tube

Rib & Lung Area

Breast

Shoulder

Lymph Nodes of Axilla

Arm

Elbow

Hip

Uterus
Rectum
Prostate

Sciatic

Ovary
Testes

Muscles of the Pelvic Region

Knee

Lymphatics of the Groin

Fallopian Tube

Appendix

Gall Bladder

Rib & Lungs

Breast Area

Elbow

Arm

Shoulder

Lymph Nodes of Axilla

Fig. 15 Reflexes on the outside of the foot

RIGHT INNER FOOT

LEFT INNER FOOT

Lymphatics of the Thigh

Lymphatics of the Groin

Fallopian Tube

Breast Area

Lungs & Ribs

Spine

Bladder

Rectum

Uterus & Prostate

Bladder

Spine

Uterus
Rectum
Prostate

Lymphatics of the Groin

Fallopian Tube

Breast Area

Lungs & Ribs

Fig. 16 Reflexes on the inside of the foot

When working on the feet of a patient, we should allow healing energy to flow through us, into our hands and into the patient. The energy of the earth comes through our feet. The energy of the universe flows through our crown chakra and both of these energies meet in the heart centre where they are united in love. From the heart this energy flows through our arms and into our hands and fingers.

When I am treating, I always start by treating the right foot and then the left. I begin by rotating the foot from the ankle joint and then rotating the toes. When doing this, care should be taken to support the joints. These simple movements help to relax the foot and the patient and to increase the flow of energy. If somebody has a stiff neck, rotating the big toe can frequently alleviate this. The position of the reflexes on the feet are as follows:

Reflexes Situated Above the Shoulder Girdle Transverse Zone

The Head Reflex   The reflexes to the head are found on all ten toes, but are duplicated on the big toe. The pad of the toe has the reflexes to the pituitary and pineal glands and the cerebellum. The reflexes to the brain are on the top and inner side of the toe, the skull along the base of the toe on top of the second phalanges, and the neck reflex is just below this. The front of the toe represents the face with the reflexes to the mouth, nose and throat.

The Spinal Reflex   This is situated along the arch of both feet. The cervical spine starts halfway along the first phalanges of the big toe and extends to the end of the second phalanges. The thoracic spine covers the length of the first metatarsal bone. The lumbar spine extends from the first cuneiform to halfway along the navicular bone. The sacrum extends to halfway along the talus and the coccyx ends part way along the calcaneus. When working with the spinal reflex, it is important to work with the reflexes to the chakras; further information on this is given in the next chapter. If a person suffers from bad headaches, I always check the coccyx. These two reflexes are related and if the coccyx has been damaged through a fall, it could cause headaches.

The Sinus Reflexes These are found on the pads of all four small toes on both feet. Work from the base of each toe to the top, including the sides and front of the toe.

The Teeth
1st incisors are on the front of the big toes.
2nd incisors and canine teeth are on the front of the second toes.
4th and 5th premolars are on the front of the third toes.
6th and 7th molars are on the front of the fourth toes.
8th molars or wisdom teeth are on the front of the fifth toes.

Arm and Shoulder Reflex Work from the elbow reflex, up the arm and into the shoulder. This is found in the fifth body zone. The arm extends along the fifth metatarsal bone into the shoulder reflex which covers the lower part of the third phalanges and extends around the side of the toe to the front.

Axillary Lymphatics These are in zone 5, on top of the foot and underneath the shoulder reflex.

Eye Reflex Found in zones 2 and 3 at the base of the second and third toes.

Ear Reflex Found in zones 3 and 4 at the base of the fourth and fifth toes.

Eustachian Tube This is situated between zones 3 and 4, between the third and fourth toes on both the tops and the soles of the feet.

Thyroid and Parathyroids This is found in zone 1, on the sole and top of the foot. The thyroid reflex covers the lower half of the second phalanges and the parathyroids are situated at the top and bottom of the inner aspect of this zone.

Reflexes Situated Between the Shoulder Girdle Transverse Zone and the Inferior Costal Margin Transverse Zone

Lung Reflex This reflex is found in zones 1 to 5 and lies between the shoulder girdle transverse zone and the diaphragm. It starts with the trachea which runs along the inner side of the cervical spine reflex, goes into the bronchus which lies underneath the thyroid reflex, opening out into the lungs.

Solar Plexus   This lies under the diaphragm, in zones 2 and 3, halfway along the second and third metatarsals.

Liver   The liver is the largest organ in the body and covers all five zones on the right foot. It lies under the diaphragm, covering the lower part of the metatarsals.

Gall Bladder   This is found on the right foot between zones 3 and 4, near the bottom of the third and fourth metatarsals. It can also be found on the top of the foot in the same position.

Oesophagus and Stomach   The oesophagus starts beneath the neck reflex in zone 1, running parallel to the spinal reflex until it joins the stomach reflex. This is found between the diaphragm and the inferior costal margin transverse zone. It covers zone 1 and part of 2 on the right foot and zones 1 to 3 on the left foot on the lower half of the metatarsal bones.

Pancreas   This coincides with part of the stomach reflex. Situated on the lower half of the metatarsals, it lies in zones 1 and 2 on the right foot and zones 1 to 3 on the left foot.

Duodenum   This is found beneath the stomach reflex, at the end of the metatarsals, covering zones 1 and 2 on the right foot and extending into zone 3 on the left foot. The inferior costal margin transverse zone runs through this reflex.

The Heart   Situated on the left foot, just above the diaphragm in zones 2 and 3.

The Spleen   To be found on the left foot in zones 4 and 5, halfway down the metatarsals.

Adrenal Glands   These lie in zone 2 towards the end of the second metatarsal bones and on top of the kidney reflex. Its close proximity to the kidney reflex can sometimes make it difficult to ascertain if a painful response is coming from the kidney or the adrenals.

Reflexes Situated Between the Inferior Costal Margin Transverse Zone and the Pelvic Floor

Bladder, Ureter Tubes and Kidneys   The bladder is found on the inner aspect of the feet, in zone 1 and at the lower end of the sacral spine. The ureter tube extends from the bladder, passing over the navicular and second cuneiform bone into zone 2 where it enters the kidney. The kidney extends just above and below the inferior costal margin transverse zone in zone 2. I feel that it is important to start working with the bladder, working up the ureter tube and into the kidney. Treating in this way clears the ureter tube, allowing any debris or small stones to pass from the kidneys into the bladder for elimination.

The Small Intestine   This is found in zones 1 to 4, just below the inferior costal margin transverse zone and extending to the top of the calcaneus.

Ileo-caecal Valve   This is situated in zone 5 at the top of the calcaneus.

The Appendix   This reflex is found on the top and the soles of the feet between the fourth and fifth zone and between the calcaneus and navicular bones.

The Large Intestine   The ascending colon on the right foot is in zone 5. It starts at the top of the calcaneus, extending to just above the inferior costal margin transverse zone. The transverse colon is situated just under the inferior costal margin transverse zone covering all five zones on the right and left feet. The descending colon is in zone 5 on the left foot, starting at the end of the fifth metatarsal and ending just below the calcaneus. The sigmoid flexure extends from zones 5 to 1, just above the calcaneus.

The Sciatic Loop   This is found a third of the way down the hard pad of the foot and extends along either side of the foot and part way up the back of the leg (Achilles tendon).

Muscles of the Pelvic Region   These cover the calcaneus on the outer aspect of both feet.

Ovaries and Testes   These reflexes are situated on the outer aspect of both feet, two-thirds up and towards the back of the calcaneus.

Fallopian Tubes From the ovaries across the talus bone on top of both feet to the inner aspect of the feet and the uterus reflex.

The Uterus and Prostate These reflexes are on the inner aspect of both feet, two-thirds up and towards the back of the calcaneus. Further reflex points for the uterus, prostate and rectum are found at the Achilles tendon at the back of the legs.

Lymphatics of the Groin and Thighs These reflexes are found on the inner and outer aspects of both feet, towards the back of the calcaneus. They go across the top of the feet, just above the reflexes to the Fallopian tubes, and up the back of the Achilles tendon.

The Hip Reflex This is in zone 5, on the outer aspect of both feet at the back of the calcaneus.

The Knee Reflex This is in zone 5, on the outer aspect of both feet following on from the hip joint to the end of the calcaneus.

Elbow Joint This is next to the knee reflex on both feet, on the inferior costal margin transverse zone.

Sacro-iliac Joint This reflex is on the outer aspect of both feet around the base of the ankle joint.

Top of the Feet

Breast Reflex This is situated in zones 2, 3 and 4 on both feet and lies in the centre of the metatarsals.

Area of the Ribs and Lungs These are found between the transverse zones of the shoulder girdle and the inferior costal margin on both feet and cover zones 1 to 5.

Upper Lymphatics and Lymph Drainage These reflexes are situated between the five toes and should be worked with at the end of a treatment.

When a treatment has been completed, I always massage both feet. I find that this relaxes the patient, especially if there has been a lot of discomfort. After this, I apply the reflexology torch, with the appropriate colour, to the reflexes which were painful.

The Spine

The human spine is a unique and very important part of the skeletal structure. It makes up about two-fifths of the total height of the body. In an average adult male, the spinal column measures about 28 inches in length and in the average adult female it measures about 24 inches.

The spine comprises seven cervical vertebrae, twelve thoracic vertebrae, five lumbar vertebrae, five sacral vertebrae and four coccygeal vertebrae. The five sacral vertebrae are fused into one bone called the sacrum and the coccygeal vertebrae are fused into one or two bones called the coccyx (Figure 17).

The spinal column could be described as a strong flexible rod that moves anteriorly, laterally and also rotates. It encloses and protects the spinal cord, supports the head and serves as a point of attachment for the ribs and the muscles of the back. Between each vertebra are openings called intervertebral foramina, through which pass the nerves that connect the spinal cord to various parts of the body.

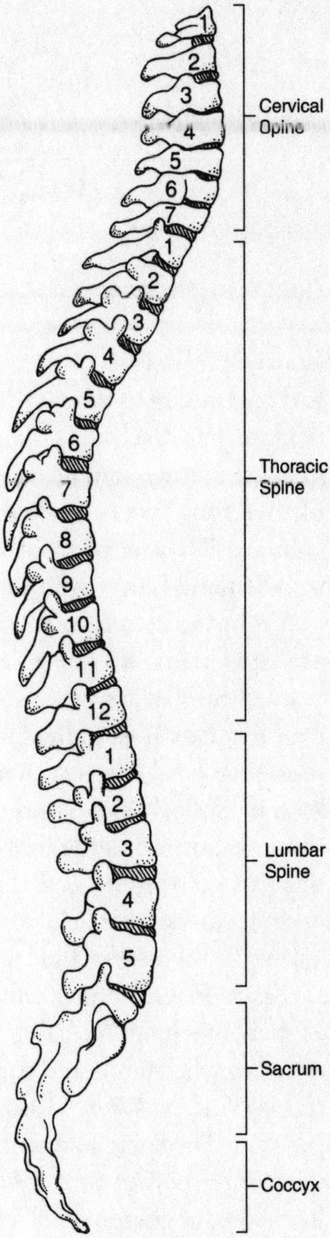

▷ **Fig. 17** The spinal column

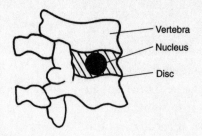

Fig. 18 An intervertebral disc

Between adjacent vertebrae, starting with the first vertebra in the neck and continuing to the sacrum, are fibrocartilaginous intervertebral discs (Figure 18). Each disc is composed of an outer fibrous ring consisting of fibrocartilage and an inner soft, pulpy elastic structure. These discs form strong joints and allow various movements of the vertebral column. They also absorb shock. Under compression they flatten, broaden and bulge from their intervertebral spaces.

From the spinal cord come thirty-one pairs of spinal nerves. There are eight pairs of cervical nerves, twelve pairs of thoracic nerves, five pairs of lumbar nerves, five pairs of sacral nerves and one pair of coccygeal nerves. The individual nerves which arise from certain regions of the spinal cord join together to form a plexus. Two plexuses are formed by the cervical nerves and one by the lumbar and sacral nerves. From these plexuses emerge individual peripheral nerves which serve different parts of the body. If there is a problem in a particular part of the body, it can be beneficial to work with the part of the spinal reflex which relates to the nerves that serve the problem area (Figure 19).

Apart from the anatomical structure and function of the spine, in esoteric teachings it is regarded as being very important. Man is the only creature who stands and walks completely upright, carrying his spine in the vertical position. Most animals carry their spine in the horizontal position. The spine in man has been referred to as 'Jacob's ladder' which we climb in order to reach higher states of consciousness. It has been likened to a golden shaft of light which grounds us to this planet but which is also capable of lifting us up into heightened awareness.

Esoteric science teaches that the spinal column houses a threefold thread. In eastern terminology these are known as the *ida*, the *pingala* and the *sushumna* paths. These three paths of life are the channels for electric fire, solar fire and fire by friction and are related in their usage to the three stages of evolution. This is part of the philosophy taught in yoga.

The kundalini fire which resides in the base chakra is the union of these three fires and will make its journey through the sushumna only when the seven main chakras or energy centres are open and a person is ready mentally, physically and spiritually. When this happens a human being is said to have reached the state of enlightenment or *samadhi* or *nirvana*.

The spinal column and its esoteric counterpart, namely the sushumna, are primarily intended to be the channel through which the energizing of the chakras and the distribution of energy to the surrounding areas of the body takes place. Failure to do this causes energy imbalances and blockages which manifest as disease in the physical body.

The metamorphic technique, discovered by Robert St John, bases its treatment on the spinal reflexes of the feet, hands and head. Robert St John believes that in the nine-month gestation period, the potentials of the human life are established. By working on the spinal reflex he believes that the prenatal period of life is brought back into focus and the life force of a person releases the energies that were impeded during this period. This allows the healing process of the body, mind and spirit to take place.

He has divided the spinal reflex into six sections (Figure 20). The first section is found on the first and second phalanges of the big toe. This is prior to the spinal reflex and represents pre-conception. The second section is situated at the first cervical vertebra and stands for conception. The third section extends from the first to the tenth thoracic vertebrae and is post-conception (1–22 weeks). The fourth section, quickening (18–22 weeks), lies between the eighth and tenth thoracic vertebrae. The fifth section, pre-birth (18–38 weeks), is found between the tenth thoracic vertebra and the coccyx, and the sixth section, birth, is located at the coccyx.

In the book *The Metamorphic Technique*, by Gaston St Pierre and Debbie Boater, it is suggested that this form of treatment should be given to a family as a whole unit as opposed to a single individual. The reason given is that metamorphic treatment can precipitate dramatic

Nerve	Innervation	Related condition
CERVICAL AREA		
1st Cervical	Blood supply to the head, pituitary, scalp, facial bones, brain, inner and middle ear, sympathetic nervous system	Headaches, nervousness, insomnia, head colds, hypertension, migraine, headaches, mental conditions, amnesia, epilepsy, tiredness, dizziness
2nd Cervical	Eyes, optic nerve, auditory nerve, sinuses, mastoid bones, tongue, forehead	Sinusitis, allergies, squint, deafness, eye troubles, earache, fainting spells, certain cases of blindness
3rd Cervical	Cheeks, outer ear, face bones, teeth, trifacial nerve	Neuralgia, neuritis, acne or pimples, eczema
4th Cervical	Nose, lips, mouth, Eustachian tube, adenoids	Hay fever, catarrh, deafness, adenoid enlargement
5th Cervical	Vocal cords, neck glands, pharynx	Laryngitis, hoarseness, pharyngitis, quinsy
6th Cervical	Neck muscles, shoulders, tonsils	Stiff neck, pain in upper arm, croup, tonsillitis, whooping cough
7th Cervical	Thyroid gland, bursa in the shoulder, the elbows	Bursitis, colds, thyroid conditions, goitre
THORACIC AREA		
1st Thoracic	Oesophagus and trachea, forearms, hands, wrists and fingers	Asthma, cough, difficult breathing, shortness of breath, pain in forearms and hands
2nd Thoracic	Heart, including its valves and covering, coronary arteries	Functional heart conditions and certain chest pains
3rd Thoracic	Lungs, bronchial tubes, pleura, chest, breast, nipples	Bronchitis, pleurisy, congestion, pneumonia, influenza
4th Thoracic	Gall bladder and common bile duct	Gall bladder conditions, jaundice, shingles
5th Thoracic	Liver, solar plexus, blood	Liver conditions, fevers, low blood pressure, anaemia, poor circulation, arthritis

Fig. 19 Nerves connected to the spine

Nerve	Innervation	Related condition
6th Thoracic	Stomach	Stomach troubles, including nervous stomach, indigestion, heart burn, dyspepsia etc.
7th Thoracic	Pancreas, islets of Langerhans, duodenum	Diabetes, ulcers, gastritis
8th Thoracic	Spleen, diaphragm	Leukaemia, hiccoughs, lowered resistance
9th Thoracic	Adrenals	Allergies, hives
10th Thoracic	Kidneys	Kidney troubles, arteriosclerosis, chronic tiredness, nephritis, pyelitis
11th Thoracic	Kidneys, urethras	Skin conditions like acne or pimples, eczema, boils, auto-intoxication
12th Thoracic	Small intestine, Fallopian tubes, lymph circulation	Rheumatism, gas pains, certain types of sterility
LUMBAR AREA		
1st Lumbar	Colon, inguinal rings	Constipation, colitis, dysentery, hernia, diarrhoea
2nd Lumbar	Appendix, abdomen, thighs, caecum	Appendicitis, cramps, difficult breathing, acidosis, varicose veins
3rd Lumbar	Sex organs, ovaries or testicles, uterus, bladder, knee	Menstrual problems like painful or irregular periods, miscarriages, impotence, menopause, bladder problems, bed-wetting, knee pains
4th Lumbar	Prostate gland, muscles of lower back, sciatic nerve	Sciatica, lumbago, difficult, painful or too frequent urination
5th Lumbar	Legs, ankles, feet, heels, arches	Poor circulation, weakness and cramps of the lower extremities, swollen ankles and arches, cold feet
THE SACRUM	Hip bones, buttocks	Sacroiliac conditions, spinal curvature
THE COCCYX	Rectum, anus	Haemorrhoids, itching, pain at end of spine on sitting

changes in an individual which can make it difficult for their family to understand and cope with the situation.

Perhaps this is another area where colour could be used to enhance the healing process.

All things that are manifest, including the colours of the spectrum, have their own vibrational frequency. The vertebrae of the spine are no exception to this. In colour therapy, Theo Gimbel uses a chart of the spine for colour diagnosis (Figure 21). He has divided the spine into four sections, each section containing eight vertebrae. Starting at the base of the spine, the first division represents the physical body, the second division the metabolic area, the third division the emotional body and the fourth division the mental body. He presents the theory that the eight flat bones of the skull are metamorphosed vertebrae and these he aligns with the spiritual aspect of a person. Each section contains the full spectrum of colour because each vertebra corresponds to the vibrational frequency of one of the spectrum colours. The colours in the part of the spine representing the physical body are dense, but as one ascends the spinal column they become lighter and more ethereal.

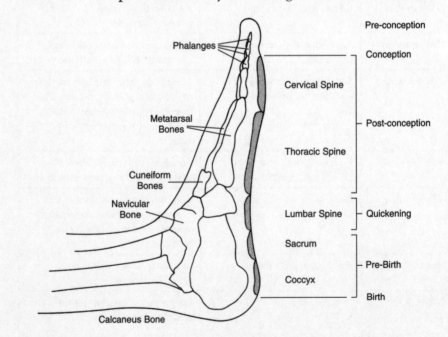

Fig. 20 Spinal reflexes of the metamorphic technique

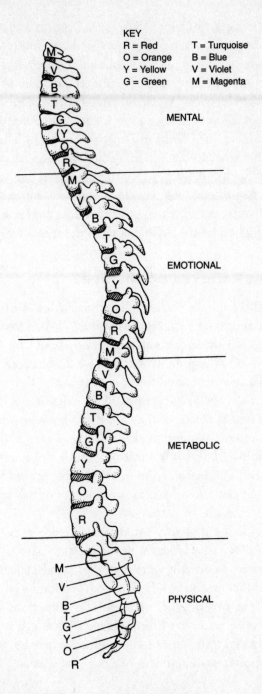

KEY
R = Red   T = Turquoise
O = Orange   B = Blue
Y = Yellow   V = Violet
G = Green   M = Magenta

MENTAL

EMOTIONAL

METABOLIC

PHYSICAL

Fig. 21 Part of the spine chart created by Theo Gimbel

In colour therapy, this spine chart is used as a colour diagnostic aid and with the help of a person's signature and a technique called dowsing, a therapist can ascertain the emotional, mental, metabolic and physical state of a patient, and also the colour and complementary colour which are needed. Working myself as a colour therapist and using this chart allows me to vouch for its authenticity. For further information on this, read *Healing Through Colour* by Theo Gimbel.

From the information that is available on the esoteric and anatomical importance of the spine, I concluded that this reflex was very important in treatment. At present I am treating a man with muscular dystrophy. He purports that the reflex which gives him the greatest sensation in his physical body, when treated with colour, is the spinal reflex.

The Chakra Reflexes on the Feet

Along the arch of the foot where the spinal reflex is situated are the reflexes to the seven main chakras (Figure 22). When treating a patient I think that it is very important that these should be worked with. Blockages in these energy centres can cause dis-harmony in the body.

The base chakra is situated towards the back of the calcaneus. The sacral chakra is where the calcaneus and navicular bones join. The solar plexus chakra is at the back of the cuneiform bone, just before it joins the navicular bone. The heart chakra is in the centre of the metatarsal bone. The throat chakra is found where the phalanges meet the metatarsal bone. The brow chakra is where the first and second phalanges meet and the crown chakra is at the top of the first phalanges, the top of the big toe.

I have found that it is very important to work with these centres during a reflexology treatment as, in the average person, one or more are out of balance. I normally work with them whilst treating the spinal reflex. If I feel that any one of them is not functioning correctly, then I spend extra time treating it. It is especially important to work with these centres if a person is suffering from a hormonal imbalance or a problem associated with one of the endocrine glands, remembering that each chakra is associated with one of these glands.

When I have completed a treatment, I then bring colour into these energy centres with the reflexology torch. If the chakras only need to be brought back into balance, then I use the dominant colour of each chakra, but if there is a physical problem in the area governed by the chakra then I would apply to the chakra the colour related to the physical problem. (See chart p.119.) For example, if a patient came in a state of hypertension, then I would administer blue to the solar plexus chakra, or if they were suffering from a 'broken heart' caused by the break-up of a relationship or a marriage, or were suffering a bereavement, then I would use violet followed by rose pink in the heart chakra. Violet or amethyst heals a broken heart and rose pink refills it with spiritual love.

Again, may I reiterate that the colours given on the chart are a foundation from which to work. Gradually learn to listen to your own intuition. It may tell you that a different colour is needed.

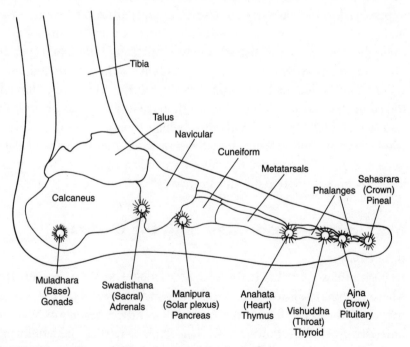

Fig. 22 The positions of the chakras on the spinal reflex

When I first started to work with colour and reflexology, I would first treat the chakras on the right foot and then on the left foot. Attending one of my workshops on reflexology and colour was a lady from Zimbabwe. At the end of these workshops I always ask participants to keep me informed on the results that they achieve using this method. This lady wrote to say that she had had some excellent results, especially when treating the chakras. She said that instead of treating the chakras on both feet separately, she had started to treat them on both feet at the same time by bringing the feet together and holding the torch between the feet at the location of the chakra. I have since tried this and found it to be very effective.

One patient that I have been working with has had a lot of emotional problems with the result that she has not had a period since the birth of her daughter three and a half years ago. After completing a normal reflexology treatment, I administered red followed by its complementary turquoise to the ovary and uterus reflexes on both feet. I then applied red to the base chakra. Her comments after this I found fascinating. She said that while I was treating the ovary and uterus reflex on the right foot, she felt as though she was still a child, the child that did not want to grow up and take responsibility. When I treated these reflexes on the left foot, she said that she felt the adult inside herself, the adult that she should be. When I then treated the base chakra, she said that she felt the child and adult being brought together to form a whole person. Interesting. Does this not show that when we treat a person, especially when we use colour, we are working with them physically, mentally, emotionally and spiritually?

Malfunctions Associated with the Chakras

Base Chakra
In yoga philosophy, this is the seat of kundalini or shakti power. It is where the union of the three subtle fires takes place: solar fire, fire by friction and electric fire. If the kundalini is raised prematurely, it can burn the protective etheric webb. This leads to nervous instability and can cause insanity.

Sacral Chakra
If this centre is not functioning properly, it can express destructive energies such as lust, anger, passion, pride and aggressiveness.

Solar Plexus Chakra
This centre is very active in the average person. It is the centre for desire and emotions. These must eventually be expressed as aspirations and raised into the heart centre. Malfunction of this chakra leads to nervousness, emotional instability, skin eruptions and hallucinations. It can promote cancer if the energies from the heart fail to find expression on the physical plane.

Heart Chakra
When this centre is correctly awakened, the energies from the solar plexus are raised to the heart chakra and expressed as love and good will. When this centre is out of balance, it can lead to heart attacks, stomach ulcers, an unhappy emotional life, fear, bitterness and resentment.

Throat Chakra
This is the creative centre, especially of the spoken word. Imbalances can be caused by sudden emotional shocks. When unbalanced it can cause asthma, vertigo, allergies, anaemia, fatigue, menstrual problems, sore throats and laryngitis.

Brow Chakra
This centre expresses idealism and imagination. When fully awake it leads to the gift of psychic powers. Imbalances lead to sinus problems, catarrh, hay fever, sleeplessness, mental stress, migraine, pessimism and self-pity.

Crown Chakra
This is the centre of higher consciousness. If this centre is opened prematurely, by the use of hallucinatory drugs, for example, then it can lead to epilepsy, coma and psychic maladjustments.

Splenic Chakra
It is through this centre that vitality is taken from the sun in the form of prana. Its incorrect function leads to depletion of energy, fatigue, depression, anaemia and lack of vitality.

CHAPTER 5

Colour

What Is Colour?

Theo Gimbel states in his book *Form, Sound, Colour and Healing* that in the beginning was the sacred darkness and out of this darkness came the light. The light and darkness danced the dance of creation and the colours of the spectrum were born.

When the sun shines after a rain storm, the rainbow appears in the sky. Through each droplet of rain this rainbow shines. If we are in the right place, we are sometimes fortunate enough to see the complete arc of shimmering translucent colours. In Genesis, Chapter 9, God makes a promise to Noah never again to destroy the earth by flood and as a sign of this promise he manifests the rainbow in the sky.

> I do set my bow in the cloud and it shall be for a token of a covenant between me and the earth.

If we look through a prism, we will see that everything that has manifested on the earth is surrounded by colour. If you have a prism, try looking through it and experience this for yourself.

Colour is most probably one of the earliest forms of therapy. Our ancestors were aware of how the colours found in nature affected them. They spent a lot of time amongst nature, absorbing and breathing in its living colours. They also realized that the colours of the foods which they ate represented another way of treating themselves.

To our ancient forefathers, colour was associated with mysticism. They knew little about the workings of the universe and to bring about harmony with the divine forces to them meant either survival or death.

Ancient civilizations regarded colour as a manifestation of the light and for this reason they related it to their deities. Likewise, Greek civilizations identified colour with universal harmony. The lives of the Egyptians were full of colour symbolism, as displayed in their art and their culture. They used the richness of colour in the charms that they wore and in their temples. Their dead they mummified and adorned with beautiful face masks and ornaments. Their priests wore breastplates of blue, symbolizing the sacredness of their judgements. Time they referred to as the everlasting green one.

All through history, colour has been associated with gods and deities. Athena, the daughter of Zeus, is reported to have worn a golden robe. To Ceres, the Roman goddess of nature, the red poppy was sacred. In Brahmanism, yellow is a sacred colour and the colour worn by the Buddha was either yellow or gold. In the Upanishads, it is written:

> In the supreme golden chamber is Brahman, invisible and pure. He is the radiant light of all lights.

The sacred colour of Mohammed is green and in Judaism, the holy colours are red, blue, purple and white.

In Atlantean times, healing was accomplished by the colours which radiated from crystals. The Atlanteans had what was known as the great healing temple. To approach the temple, one had to climb a flight of twelve steps and pass between twelve columns, six on either side, before entering into the large circular room. The ceiling of the temple was domed and created out of interlocking crystals which displayed all the colours of the spectrum. These crystals formed patterns of ancient symbols and when the light shone through the dome, it created exquisite patterns of colour and vibration. Around the circumference of this room were individual healing rooms used for many purposes, for example, for before and after childbirth, for specific ailments and diseases, and in assisting the transition of a soul from this life to the next.

In ancient times, gems were used in Ayurvedic medicine because they were looked upon as a condensation of the seven cosmic rays. Seven main gems were used for the seven main colours. These were ruby (red), pearl (orange), coral (yellow), emerald (green), topaz (blue), diamond (indigo) and sapphire (violet). These gems were always examined through a prism to ascertain their true cosmic colour, as their users believed that the manifested colour was not always the true colour essence of the stone. Apart from these main seven, two others were used. These were onyx, which they believed radiated the ultraviolet ray, and cat's-eye for the infra-red ray. These gems were made into medicine in two ways. They were either burnt to ashes and the ash administered to the patients, or the gems were kept in alcohol for seven days so that the alcohol could absorb the vibrations of the gems. Gemstones are still used in this way in Ayurvedic medicine.

Today, colour is again becoming one of the important complementary therapies. If you like, it is being rediscovered. Having said this, how does it work?

From reading the chapter on the electromagnetic spectrum, we can understand that each of the colours of the spectrum has its own vibration. Therefore, by using colour on its own or in conjunction with another therapy, we can maintain or alter the vibrations of the body to a frequency which induces health and harmony.

All things manifested in the universe have their own vibration. Likewise, each cell, organ, muscle and bone in the human body vibrates to a set frequency. If this frequency changes, it causes dis-ease. The cause for these changes are many but I believe that the greatest cause is stress. This is prevalent in the society in which we live. We are so busy trying to cope with the pressures of day-to-day living that we, unlike our ancestors, no longer have time to stop, relax and absorb the wonderful colours which nature has given us.

If one of the cells of our body is at the wrong frequency, it affects its electromagnetic field. This will then affect the force field of the related organ, eventually spreading to affect the auric field surrounding us. If we introduce back into this organ the correct vibration through the frequency of colour, we can rebalance its altered function. The body always has the tendency to revert back to its original pattern, given the right conditions.

Like our manifested physical body, each of our auric bodies has its own frequency of vibration. If one of these bodies is vibrating at the wrong frequency, then the rest are affected. Everything that we do affects our aura and if what we are doing is detrimental, then an imbalance in the vibration occurs. This changes its colour and reflects itself in the endocrine glands, nervous system and organs of the physical body.

It is a known fact that the mind affects the body and the body affects the mind. Thinking about our mind and the thought patterns which are created, can we attribute colour to these thoughts? If so, are we not inflicting detrimental colours upon ourselves and our environment with negative thoughts and beneficial healing colours with positive thoughts? I know that it is not always easy to think positively, but, with practice, it can be achieved. One of the ways to create healing colours in our thought patterns is with colour meditations. These have been included in this book, together with the explanation of each colour, for you to work with.

Colour is being used as a therapy in many different ways. Remembering that our body is light-sensitive, colour can be transmitted through the use of stained glass onto the body of a person or it can be applied to the body through crystals. Working myself with colour therapy, I have chosen to use it in contact healing. To be able to do this, one has to sensitize the most perfect instrument which we have, namely the human body, and open this up as a pure channel for the colours of the universe to flow through. If one is training to become a colour therapist, this technique is part of the training. One also learns how to visualize and to feel colour. The length of time that this takes depends upon the sensitivity of the person concerned but, with regular practice, it can be achieved. The next chapter explains techniques which will enable you to sensitize your own beautiful instrument so that if you prefer, you can administer colour to the reflex zones of your patient through yourself instead of through the reflexology torch.

Having trained as a colour therapist as well as a reflexologist and realizing that our auric bodies as well as each cell, organ, gland, bone and muscle in our physical body has its own vibrational frequency which relates to one of the colours of the spectrum, I started to apply colour to the painful reflex zones after a normal reflexology treatment. I was surprised at the very positive results that I got. When I use colour in this way, I always apply the colour required followed by its complementary. This applies only to the zones on the feet and not to the chakras. It has been shown, through the work of Theo Gimbel, that if only the treatment colour is used, the change in the vibrational frequency is not constant. He gives the example of treating high blood pressure with blue. He states that during the treatment the blood pressure fell, but a short time after the treatment it rose again dramatically. He then treated with blue and its complementary orange and found that by doing this, the blood pressure remained constant after the treatment. Inside the back cover the colours are given with their complementary colours.

Let us now explore ways in which the body can be sensitized to colour before looking at the individual colours, the diseases which they are used to treat and how these colours are applied to the zones of the feet.

Sensitizing the Body to Colour

Each one of us has the potential to be a channel for healing. Whether or not we choose to do so is up to us. If we choose to do so it can cause dramatic changes in our lives, old patterns being broken down in order that new ones may be formed, which is frequently a very uncomfortable process. We have to learn to flow with the energies, not knowing where they are leading us. Through this experience we have to learn to trust in the Divine Being, God, Buddha, Universal Intelligence, whatever name one calls this supreme power. If we dedicate ourselves as channels, we have to trust that we will be looked after and given what we need when it is needed. If we are working for the universe and the good of our fellow human beings, I can assure you that we are looked after and provided for. Learn to live in the now, realizing that we cannot relive or be remorseful about the past. We can only look at it, remember the positive things and be thankful for what our mistakes have taught us. We can plan for the future but it may never come. Tomorrow we may die or the world may come to an end. What have we got left? The Now.

Yogic philosophy teaches that all things are now. Enlightenment is now, eternity is now. Being a channel for healing starts now.

To dedicate oneself to this life style involves discipline. Part of this discipline is meditation, tuning in to our inner tuition, our higher self, the divine part of us that knows the answers to all things. We have to learn to listen and to trust. In some ways we have to learn to live a 'schizophrenic' existence, learning to tune in and become one with the higher powers of the universe but at the same time be fully grounded on this earth plane, carrying out the duties and responsibilities we have undertaken. How true is the saying that in being too heavenly minded we are no earthly good. We incarnated onto this planet in order to evolve and to learn. We came here with various tasks to accomplish, various hurdles to jump over. When confronted with these, again we have the choice as to whether we go over them or leave them for the next time round. I always liken this earth plane to a school of learning. When we have finished what we came to learn and accomplish, we go home for a holiday.

Once we have decided to become a channel for healing, how do we start? We have said that it involves discipline, part of which is meditation, but what next?

We have to learn to know ourselves. To know our physical body and to sensitize and raise its vibrational frequency. Here I am reminded of part of the Anglican liturgy for Ash Wednesday:

Oh man, know thyself and the place from which thou comest.

We can become a good, bad or mediocre channel. How good or bad we are depends upon the state of our body, physically, mentally and emotionally. If we use a hosepipe to channel water, it has to be clean and clear to produce a strong and steady flow. If it is twisted or clogged up, the stream of water passing through it will not be adequate. This also applies to us. If we are constantly worried, under stress, allowing our mind to rule us, this interferes with the flow of energy. If our emotional body is unstable and we allow ourselves to over-react and become emotionally involved with other people's problems as well as our own, again we are causing blockages within ourselves. If we do not take care of our physical body and create harmony within ourselves by giving ourselves enough rest, the right kind of food, enough exercise and adequate daylight, our body will not serve us well and will not be clear enough to channel the finer energies of healing.

In the *Bhagavad Gita*, Chapter 6, verse 16, it says:

Yoga is a harmony,
Not for him who eats too much or for
    him who eats too little.
Not for him who sleeps too little, not for
    him who sleeps too much.

A harmony in eating and resting, in
   sleeping and keeping awake.
A perfection in whatever one does.
This is the yoga that gives peace from all pain.

Many of us have abused and taken our physical body so much for grant-
ed that we are no longer aware of it. We only notice it if there is pain
and disorder. We then run to the doctor and resort to drugs which have
side effects, creating further disharmony, in order to relieve the symp-
tom. Very few of us take the time to stop and listen to our body in an
endeavour to find out the cause of the disharmony, to find out what
we are doing that is wrong. In order to be able to do this successfully,
we need to become aware and in tune with ourselves.

Let us start by doing a very simple relaxation exercise.

♦ Find a place which is quiet and warm and where you will not be
disturbed. If you need to, take the receiver off the telephone. Find
yourself a blanket to cover yourself and a pillow to place under your
head. When the body starts to relax, the metabolic rate slows down
and the body becomes cold. Remove or loosen any tight clothing.

Lie down on the floor. Place the pillow beneath your head and
cover yourself with the blanket. Make sure that your body is straight
with your legs slightly apart. Place your hands on the floor, palms
facing upwards, about 6 inches away from the body. Tuck your chin
into your chest so that the cervical (neck) part of your spine is straight.

Try to free your mind of all unnecessary and worrying thoughts.
As these thoughts enter your mind, look at them and then visualize
them as beautiful bubbles. Allow them to float up into the atmosphere where they gently disperse. As your mind becomes quieter
and still, bring your concentration into your physical body.

First concentrate on your feet. Try to visualize the bones, muscles, flesh and skin which form your feet. Feel for any tension in
your feet. Gently let go of this tension, allowing your feet to become
very heavy and relaxed.

Move up both of your legs. Feel your ankles, calves, shins, knees
and thighs. Visualize the bones and muscles which are contained in
your legs. Feel for any tension. As you let go of this tension, feel
your legs becoming very heavy and relaxed.

From your legs, move up into your abdomen. Experience not only the skeletal structure and the muscles supporting this but also the organs contained in this part of your body. If you do not know about the anatomy of your body, read about it, learn how your body works. By doing this and becoming aware of what is happening to it, you will be conscious when things start to go wrong and learn how to put them right, bringing the body back into harmony. Feel for any tension in your abdomen. If there is tension, release it. Allow your abdomen to relax and to become very heavy. Try to remember that tension not only affects the muscles of the body but all the organs and systems as well.

From your abdomen, move into your solar plexus. This is a place where a lot of tension can accumulate and be felt due to the ganglia of nerve endings here. Try to be aware of any tension or anxiety in this part of your body. Relax. Let go of all tension. It is not part of you and you do not need it.

Move up into your chest. Feel the gentle inhalation and exhalation of the breath, the slow rhythmic beat of your heart. Visualize your ribcage and the muscles which surround it. With each exhalation, release any tension in this part of your body. Your heart is a muscular organ and is also prone to tension.

From your chest move across your shoulders, down both of your arms, into your hands and fingers. Visualize any tension in this part of your being as a grey mist which floats out into the atmosphere and disperses, leaving your hands, arms and shoulders relaxed and heavy.

Lastly, come into your neck and head. Relax your throat and all the muscles surrounding your neck. Relax your tongue, your jaws, your eyes, forehead, the top and back of your head. Allow your neck and head to become very heavy and relaxed.

Lastly, feel the whole of your body, which should now be in a state of complete relaxation. Consciously go through your body and if you find any place where there is still tension, relax it.

Stay in this state of relaxation, peace and tranquillity for fifteen minutes. If it helps, you can play music during this time, making sure that the tape is long enough to last from the beginning to the end of your relaxation.

When your fifteen minutes have ended, slowly start to come out of relaxation. Start by gently moving your toes, then rotating your ankles, flexing the muscles in your legs, moving your fingers as if playing a piano keyboard. Then, breathing in, raise your arms over your head, stretching your whole body. Breathing out, bring your hands back to the floor. Repeat this twice more. Slowly move your head from side to side, then when you are ready, open your eyes, roll over onto your right side and sit up.

Sit still for a few minutes and try to be aware of any changes that may have taken place within you. These changes could be mental, emotional or physical. If you would like to, you could keep a notebook on your progress.

Try to do this relaxation exercise every day. In doing this you will begin to be aware of yourself and instinctively know what your body does and does not need. Try to set aside the same time each day, as this provides a discipline which you should find easier to follow.

After practising this for two to three weeks, you should be ready to move on to the next stage. Having become acquainted with and aware of your physical body, the next step is to try to feel your aura or electromagnetic field which surrounds you.

◆ Lie down on the floor and go into relaxation as described in the previous exercise.

When your body and mind are in a state of peace and relaxation, bring your concentration into the inhalation and exhalation of the breath. With each exhalation, feel your awareness expanding until it fills the room in which you are lying. In this state, try to feel your seven main energy centres or chakras. Start with the base or muladhara. Move into the sacral or swadisthana, the solar plexus or manipura, the heart or anahata, the throat or vishuddha, the brow or ajna, and finally to the crown or sahasrara.

The sensation felt at these energy centres varies with individuals. Some people feel heat or cold, others a vibration and a few the sensation of pain. You have to recognize your own sensation for these chakras. If at first you feel nothing, do not be disappointed. Sensitizing the body takes time and it is important that you work at the speed which is right for you.

Whether you can or cannot feel these centres, try to visualize yourself lying in the middle of a rainbow. The colours nearest to your physical body are dense, gradually getting paler and more ethereal the further away they are from you. Try to step outside this scene and look to see if you can discern where each colour radiates from.

Practise this for five to ten minutes and then return from this visualization and relaxation as described earlier. Again, practise this exercise for a couple of weeks before moving on.

The third part of this exercise continues where part two ended.

♦ Having consciously stepped aside from your physical body to look at and feel the chakras, the next stage is to try to feel each individual chakra and colour. This exercise starts by putting the body into relaxation, then stepping aside from the body. Try to feel and locate the base chakra. Allow yourself to enter this centre. Feel the colour red which emanates from it. What sensation does the vibrational frequency of this colour give you? How do you react to it? Slowly move through the remaining six chakras, feeling the vibrational frequency of the colours and the effect they have upon you.

When you have completed this, slowly start to come out of relaxation. Gently open your eyes and digest what you have experienced.

♦ When you next practise this exercise, at the end, after sitting up, bring your concentration into the palms of your hands. Remember that in the palm of each hand is a minor chakra. Raise your hands so that the palms are about 4 inches apart, facing each other. Close your eyes and try to feel an energy building up between your two palms; visualize this as a white ball of light. As this light grows, move your hands further apart. If you practise this in a darkened room, you may be able to see this energy as a white glowing light. Now place this energy onto any part of your body where there is discomfort and feel it establishing harmony and peace. If this exercise is practised with a friend, you can give this energy to each other. Later on, when you understand and know the meaning of the colours, you can infuse your ball of light energy with the colour needed by yourself or your friend.

For the next exercise, you will need eight pieces of natural material, either cotton or silk. Each piece should be dyed with one of the ten colours of the spectrum.

◆ Find yourself a quiet, warm place and sit either on the floor or on a chair, placing your pieces of material on the floor beside you. Taking one colour at a time, place the material on the palm of your left hand. Hold the palm of your right hand about 6 inches above the material. Close your eyes and try to feel through the chakra in your right hand the vibrational frequency of each colour. Make a note of what you experience.

If you work with a partner, you can close your eyes, allowing your partner to place a colour onto your hand. You then have to guess which colour you are holding.

After each colour, lay the energy of that colour to the elements before moving on to the next colour. To do this, place your hands onto the ground, palms downwards and say:

Earth to earth,
Water to water,
Fire to fire,
Air to air.

If this is not done, the vibrations of each colour will mingle and you will not be able to discern one from the other.

Coloured material can be worn in the form of clothes in order to introduce the correct vibrational frequencies into our body to restore it to harmony. For example, if you are suffering from a sore throat, a silk turquoise scarf worn round your neck will help. If you are depressed, a bright orange blouse or skirt will help to lift you out of your depression. A blue dress will help if you are under stress. If you are wearing coloured garments to help to bring your body back into harmony, remember to wear white underneath. Otherwise, the colours of the outer garment and the inner garment will blend when daylight passes through them and the colour that you will receive will be a combination of the two.

From using coloured material, you can move on to other living colours found in flowers, grasses, trees and birds. Nature is full of the most beautiful colours displayed in every shade imaginable. As you become more sensitive to colour, you cannot help becoming more aware of nature.

Let us use nature for our next awareness exercise. For this you will need access to a garden or a place where there is grass. It needs to be a dry day and relatively warm.

♦ With bare feet, go outside and walk on the grass. Notice the action of your feet in walking, how they are placed onto the grass and how they are taken off to enable you to walk forward. Try to feel if one part of your foot is more sensitive than the rest. Feel to see if the temperature of the grass is uniform or whether it changes. After a little while, stand still and, remembering that you have a minor chakra on the sole of each foot, try to feel the colour of the grass through these. Feel this colour flooding your feet and rising up your legs into your trunk, arms, hands and head. Feel any toxins being removed from your body and the positive and negative energies being brought into balance. Continue to walk very slowly over the grass. Take note to see if your feet have become more sensitive to touch. Are you able to feel more than when you first started? Do this for as long as you feel comfortable.

When we work with colour, either as a colour therapist or in conjunction with reflexology, we need to learn to visualize as well as sensitize our body to colour. There is a very thin line between visualization and imagination. To begin with, most people use imagination. Imagination is when you know what an object looks like, for example a yellow daffodil, and when you close your eyes and recall what you know about this flower, you get an imaginary picture of it (Figure 23). Visualization is when you look at a daffodil, close your eyes and actually see it in front of your closed eyes.

The easiest way to experience visualization for yourself is with a lighted candle (Figure 24).

♦ Sit in a dark room and place the lighted candle in front of you. Bring all of your concentration into the flame and stare into it until your eyes start to water. Then close your eyes. You should see in front of your closed eyes the flame of the candle. It will most probably move around, eventually going out of focus. It is only with practice that we are able to keep it still and in focus.

Why do we need to visualize? If we are bringing colour through ourselves we need to visualize the colour that we wish to flow through our hands and into the patient. Sometimes, especially if we have sensitized our body to colour, we become aware that a different colour from the one we visualized is being projected through us. This is correct and we should allow it to happen. Remember, if we have dedicated ourselves as an instrument, the higher powers know better than we what colour a person needs.

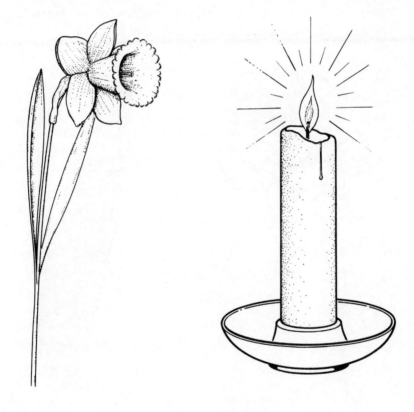

Fig. 23   **Fig. 24**

♦ For this next visualization exercise, you will need a single flower of your choice and colour (Figure 25). Put it into a vase and place the vase in front of you. Direct all of your attention onto that flower. Observe how it is formed, how many petals it has, whether or not the petals are all the same. If not, what are the variations? Look at the colour of the flower. Is this the same throughout or are some parts of the flower lighter in colour?

Now take the flower and very gently place it onto the palm of your left hand. Place the right hand about 4 inches above it. Close your eyes and try to feel through the palm of your right hand the colour which it emanates. Place the flower back into the vase and again close your eyes but this time, try to visualize the flower before your closed eyes. If you have been keeping a notebook on your experiences, write down what you did or did not feel.

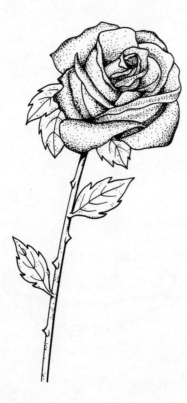

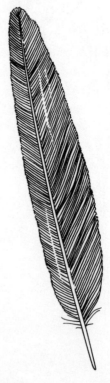

Fig. 25   **Fig. 26**

This sensitivity exercise can be done with stones, leaves, feathers (Figure 26) or crystals. When working with these things, remember that they all contain life, even the humble stone that you pick up on the path. Its vibrational rate is very slow but it is living. Try to have respect and love for all of nature and in return it will reward you.

When we work as a channel for colour healing, we work not only with colour but also with the earth energies and the spiritual energies. The earth energies come through our feet into the heart chakra and the spiritual energies enter through our crown chakra into the heart. Here they are united in love before radiating down our arms and into our hands and fingers. If we use colour, we bring the red, orange, gold and yellow rays up from the earth, spring green and emerald enters horizontally into the heart chakra, and the blue, indigo, violet and magenta enter through the top of our head.

For this last exercise, we are going to try to channel the healing energies and the colour through ourselves into our hands.

◆ Find a place which is quiet and warm and where you will not be disturbed. Either sit on the floor or on a chair, whichever you find more comfortable. Mentally go through your body, releasing any tension. Now bring your concentration to the inhalation and exhalation of the breath. With each exhalation, breathe out any negativity or tension still remaining. Feel your metabolism slowing down and a sense of peace and tranquillity pervading your being.

The colour which you are going to channel is blue. Concentrate on this colour and try to visualize it. If you find it helpful, start by imagining a blue object or flower. When you have done this, visualize a shaft of blue light entering your crown chakra and descending into the heart centre. Be also aware of the earth and spiritual energies meeting here. Concentrate on these three energies being united by love, then allow this combined energy to flow down your arms and into your hands. Visualize your hands becoming infused with blue light. If any part of your body is tense or aching, place your fingers onto it and visualize this blue light passing out of your fingers and into the chosen area of your body.

Now relax for a moment and recollect any thoughts or sensations that you may have experienced.

This exercise can be practised using any of the ten colours but do read the meaning of the colours and what specific ailment each colour is used for before doing this. You might like to channel it through your fingers and into the reflex zones on your feet. If you do this, may I suggest that you start with blue and channel it into the solar plexus.

At the beginning of this chapter, I mentioned that meditation is part of the discipline required if we wish to become a channel for healing. I therefore feel that it is important to mention something about this before embarking upon the individual colours and their properties.

CHAPTER 6
Guidelines for Meditation

Meditation is a discipline, a discipline which teaches us to relax the body and quieten the mind in order to contact the divine spark or true self within us, that part of us which has no beginning and no ending.

When we first start on the path of meditation, many difficulties are encountered. The first is disciplining ourselves to set aside time each day to practise. The second is learning to sit still and to relax the body, and the third is quieting the mind, which most people find extremely difficult to do. Under normal circumstances, our mind rules us. We are now endeavouring to reverse this and become master over our mind. Like a spoilt child, the mind rebels as soon as we sit down to meditate and bombards us with thoughts on every subject we care to name. Patanjali, a wise eastern sage, likens the mind to a pond into which is thrown a continuous stream of stones, which cause ripples upon the pond's surface. The pond represents the mind, the stones thoughts and the ripples the disturbances that these thoughts cause. Unless we stop throwing stones, allow the ripples to cease and the surface of the pond to become still, we will never see the bottom. In other words, if we are unable to quieten the mind and free it from thoughts we will never realize our own true self, the eternal flame within us.

There are many ways of practising mind control. One can achieve this through mantras (the repetition of special sounds), yantras (geometric forms), concentration on the breath, listening to music, imagery and many other techniques. I found the best thing to do was to investigate all of the techniques and then select the one which gave me the best results.

If you meditate in a group, it is advisable to start with guided meditation. This allows the group to become familiar with each other's vibrations in order to create harmony. This could take six to eight weeks. When this has been achieved, it is then possible for the group to go into silence.

If you meditate alone, you may find it helpful to keep a spiritual diary. In this, you write down what you have achieved, learnt and experienced through each meditation.

Another aspect which can be included in meditation is absent healing. Once the mind is quiet and we have achieved a higher level of consciousness, we can lift those souls who have asked for absent healing into the light. We can visualize them lying in a beautiful garden and mentally project to them the colours which they need. Another way is to visualize a temple of healing into which you take these people. Here, they can either be given the water of life, healing and health, or else infused with the colours which flood these temples.

When we start to practise meditation, it is important that the same time is set aside each day. This then becomes a discipline creating a good habit. It is so easy to have the good intention to practise each day and, if a fixed time is not set aside, the day passes, evening comes and we feel too tired to do our meditation.

When you meditate, find a place which is quiet and warm and where you will not be disturbed. If necessary, take the telephone off the hook. This is a very special time which you have created for yourself and your own inner development. Light a candle and dedicate it to the Christ light, the Buddha light or to whatever path or deity you follow. If you sit on a chair, sit in the Pharaoh posture, with both feet on the floor, hands resting on your knees, the palms either facing down or up. If they face down, it is symbolic of receiving and if they face up it symbolizes giving. Your spine should be straight, your head and neck relaxed and your eyes closed. If you are sitting on the floor, you can sit against the wall with your legs out straight, in full or half lotus or in simple crossed leg posture. Again, it is important that your spine is straight. Remember that your spine is like a golden shaft of light which earths you to this planet but which is also able to lift you up into the higher realms of consciousness.

Try to let go of any thoughts which come into your mind. Visualize them as beautiful bubbles which float up into the atmosphere and gently disperse. When your mind has become quiet and still, bring your concentration into your physical body. Go through your body, releasing any tension in the organs and muscles. If your body feels uncomfortable, change its position. Now that your body and mind is quiet and still, proceed with your chosen meditation.

In meditation, we are working with the seven main chakras or energy centres. These are the gateways which lead us into the higher states of consciousness and they open when we are in a meditative state. It is therefore of the utmost importance that we close them at the end of each meditation. If this is not done, we are leaving open doors through which unwelcome entities can enter. The most effective way to close them is to visualize a cross of light enclosed within a circle of light (Figure 27) and, starting with the crown, place this symbol around each of the seven main chakras. Visualize this as a golden key which securely locks each of these centres of higher perception.

▷ **Fig. 27** A cross of light within a circle of light used as a golden key to close all the centres of higher perception

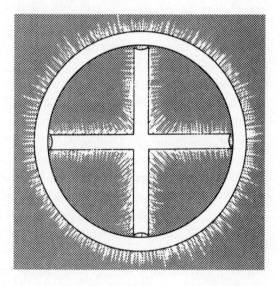

When you have completed this, start to increase your inhalation and exhalation. Become aware of your physical body sitting either on the floor or on a chair. Then, when you are ready, gently open your eyes and be fully returned to earth consciousness.

Extinguish the candle and send the light either to somebody who is in need of healing or to any troubled part of the world. Be thankful for any experience or insight which has been given to you.

If you find difficulty in concentrating or quieting your mind, do not be discouraged. These things only come with practice. Some days you may have no difficulty and your meditation is a beautiful experience. On other days you may find it very hard and spend the whole time trying to concentrate and still your mind. Do not give up if this happens. All of the experiences which we are given help to strengthen us. If your mind constantly wanders, gently bring it back. With regular practice and perseverance, meditation will become an essential part of your life.

The Elementals

When walking in the countryside or working with the gifts that nature has given to us, I feel that it is important to acknowledge and work with the elementals who are responsible for the elements of earth, water, fire and air. If we ask their help and thank them for helping us, they will become our friends and servants. If we misuse them, they can create havoc.

The elementals pertaining to the earth kingdom are the gnomes, to the water kingdom, the undines, to the fire kingdom, the salamanders, and to the kingdom of air, the sylphs.

I remember, a long time ago, hearing a programme on the radio where a lady was interviewed who claimed that she had seen fairies at the bottom of her garden. She was laughed at and purported to be eccentric. Was she eccentric or was she gifted in being able to see these beings? I know that many of the people who work at Findhorn with the elementals claim to have seen them. Findhorn, in Scotland, is where a community of people live and work together. They have grown what could be termed as prize vegetables in soil which the average gardener would regard as unsuitable. They are reputed to have achieved this by enlisting the help of the elementals and devas associated with the plant kingdom.

This meditation includes these beings and in it we thank them for the tasks they are accomplishing.

Morning Meditation

Before starting this meditation, read the instructions given on pages 78–9.

♦ Imagine that you are standing at the end of a narrow and dimly lit corridor. Slowly you start to walk down this corridor. You feel the unevenness of the floor beneath your feet and you notice that the walls are made of rock which is rough and jagged to touch. The further down the corridor you walk, the dimmer becomes the light but there is enough light for you to distinguish the door which you are approaching. It is made from wood and has a round wooden handle on its right-hand side. You take hold of the handle, sensing the smoothness and warmth of the wood and turn it, opening the door outwards.

As you walk through the doorway, you find yourself in the countryside. It is still dark and everything is still and silent. Lifting your gaze to the sky, you look into a star-bespeckled bowl which twinkles and shines like hundreds of precious jewels. The bright crescent moon is surrounded by a luminous aura.

Starting to walk along the path that you find yourself standing on, you feel the stones and gravel beneath your feet. Some feel smooth, others sharp. You remember with gratitude the elementals who are responsible for the mineral kingdom, the gnomes. In remembering these elementals, your thoughts turn to the beautiful crystals which are formed in the darkness of the earth, the white of the diamond through to the violet of the amethyst. You are reminded that out of the sacred darkness comes light.

Stepping off this gravel path and onto the grass, you feel through your feet the difference in texture. The grass feels smooth and soft, with a slightly colder sensation. You become aware that different parts of your feet pick up different sensations. Stop for a moment and look at the might and majesty of the surrounding trees, still clothed in the mist of night. They seem to be inviting you to share the energy that they absorbed during the day. As you stand and look with awe and wonder, the sound of distant water reaches you. Its rippling, bubbling music invites you to walk towards it. The sound grows louder as you approach the brook whose waters dance their way across the countryside. On its banks is tethered a boat. Get into it and allow the brook to carry you along with it. Lying back in the boat, you sense that dawn is just about to break. Behind you, the sky is still a deep indigo, but as you move your gaze towards the horizon, the indigo turns into a pale blue. Placing your hand over the side of the boat and into the water, you feel a tingling coldness. The water seems to wash away any tension in your hand, leaving it relaxed and refreshed. Gliding gently along, you remember with thankfulness the elementals who are responsible for the element of water, the undines.

Slowly your boat drifts into a small bay and stops. You get out and secure it to a mooring post.

The sun is now rising over the horizon and dawn has almost broken. In front of you grows a beautiful magnolia tree, laden with white and magenta blossom. You sit beneath its boughs, absorbing its colours into your being, and breathe in its delicate perfume. A gentle breeze softly rustles its leaves and plays around your face and hair. It reminds you of the elementals who are responsible for the element of air, the sylphs, and you thank them.

Dawn has now fully broken and the sun glows a golden orange on the horizon. Farm animals and birds have awakened to this new day and sing and call to each other. The noise of farmhands starting their work travels across the countryside. You feel the warmth from the newly risen sun radiating on your body and energizing every cell and atom. In thankfulness you remember the salamanders, the elementals who are responsible for the element of fire. Your whole being starts to radiate peace, tranquillity and love.

Realizing that it is time to return from this peace and solitude, slowly stand up and look around you. You notice that the boat in which you travelled brought you in almost a complete circle and just a few yards in front of where you are sitting is the door through which you came.

You stand up and walk to the door, turn the handle and open the door towards you. Walk through it, back into the corridor. After the brilliance of the dawn, the corridor seems very dark and narrow. Continue to walk along the corridor until you enter the room where you started this meditation.

Become aware of your body. Slowly start to increase your inhalation and exhalation. Now close down your centres of higher perception as instructed on page 79 and be fully returned to earth consciousness.

The Rainbow Meditation

Prepare yourself for this meditation by following the instructions given on pages 78–9.

♦ Imagine yourself standing at the end of a corridor. There is very little light, but you are able to discern that the walls are composed of natural stone, rough and uneven and the floor is made up of cobbles. They feel smooth and cold to your bare feet. Looking down the corridor, you see at its end a shaft of golden light. Slowly you start to walk towards it. The nearer you get, the brighter it becomes. It seems to be beckoning you. As you approach this light, you find that it is shining through a partly opened door. Taking hold of the edge of the door, you open it and find that you are standing at the entrance to a circular room.

Walking into the room, you discover that you have walked into a giant rainbow. Each colour of this rainbow ascends from the outer edges of the floor, meeting near the centre of the ceiling. Stand and look at this spectacle with awe and wonder. The colours of red, orange, yellow, green, turquoise, blue, violet and magenta are shimmering and dancing with life. Their individual energies are alive and each colour conveys to you a message.

Slowly start to walk around the perimeter of the room. As you do this, the first colour that you walk into is red. You feel its warmth penetrating your body, its energy grounding you to this planet.

Moving forward, you become surrounded by the orange ray. It takes away from you any depression or heaviness that you may be feeling and it replaces it with joy and laughter. You allow this colour to energize every cell and atom of your body.

From orange, you pass into yellow and you feel yourself becoming detached. Detached from emotional and physical problems, detached from people and acquaintances. From this state of detachment, you find that you are able to view your life from a new perspective. You are shown the various paths which you can take to overcome any physical and/or emotional problems that you may be experiencing. You can look at your friends and relations and realize that what they are doing and experiencing is for their own inner growth, not to be judged or criticized but to be watched with love, knowing that you will always be ready and happy to extend a loving, helping hand when needed.

Walk out of the yellow and into the green. Stop and experience what this colour is doing for you. Feel it removing all toxins from your body and bringing your positive and negative energies into balance. Ask this colour to bring the three aspects of your being, body, mind and spirit, into harmony so that you may become whole or holy.

Leaving this colour, you enter the energy of blue. Immediately you feel all of the tension in your body being released and replaced by a deep sense of peace and tranquillity. In comparison to the red ray, the blue feels cool to your body.

Taking this sense of peace and tranquillity with you, walk on into the violet ray. Violet, the colour of dignity. Allow it to give you that dignity which you should have as a human being, dignity in the physical, emotional and mental aspects of your being.

Lastly, walk on into the magenta ray. Let this colour dissolve all old emotional, metabolic, mental and physical patterns which are no longer right for you, old patterns which must be dissolved in order that you can grow and evolve into the next stage of your inner development.

Feeling that these colours have stripped you of your old raiment and dressed you with new, walk through the magenta ray into the centre of the rainbow.

At the centre, you find yourself in pure white light. Looking up to the centre of the ceiling, you discover that this white light is formed by all the colours merging into one. The one pure light of God consciousness.

On the floor in the centre of this pillar of light is a round, shallow pond. Upon it water lilies float and around its edges are crystals of all shapes, sizes and colours. There are rubies, amber, yellow topaz, emeralds, turquoise, sapphires and amethysts. Sit down by the side of this pond and try to sense which crystal is asking you to come and hold it. Find that crystal and then, taking it into your hands, feel its energy through your hands. Ask it to reveal to you where it came from. This may come in the form of pictures which appear before your inner eye or from your own inner tuition. Now take the crystal and place it against any part of your body which needs healing. Allow its energy to bring that part of your body back into harmony. With gratitude and love, place the crystal back by the side of the pond.

You now realize that it is time to leave the centre of this beautiful rainbow and return once more to earth consciousness.

Turn in the opposite direction from which you entered the centre of this rainbow and walk out through the red ray. As you walk through this ray, you feel the colour of red returning and grounding you once more to this planet. Walking out of this ray, go through the door and back into the corridor. Walk down the corridor until you come back into the room where you started this meditation. Be aware of your body sitting on the floor or chair and gently start to return to everyday activity, remembering to close down your centres of higher perception as instructed on page 79.

This next meditation is used for those people who have asked for absent healing. It is a good idea to have a notebook where you can keep a list of these people's names. It is so easy to forget someone. This book can be kept either in your healing room or where you practise your meditation.

Absent-healing Meditation

Prepare yourself for meditation by following the instructions given on pages 78–9.

♦ Try to visualize a beautiful temple, round in structure, with a domed roof. This roof is created out of interlocking crystals which, as the sun shines through them, fill the temple with rainbows of light. In the centre of the temple is a fountain, the fountain of life, light and harmony. Around the circumference of the temple are doors behind which are individual healing rooms. Each room is flooded with an individual colour of the spectrum.

In this temple the elders gather to help those who are seeking their path or who have come for healing. There are also those souls who have just completed their life on earth and those who are waiting to incarnate.

Standing quietly by the fountain, visualize all those who have asked for healing coming and standing with you in the temple. By the side of the fountain are cups. Take one of these and fill it with water from the fountain. First you drink of this water of life, light and harmony and then you offer the cup to those who have come for healing. As they drink, visualize their body, mind and spirit being brought into harmony and their whole being radiating health and peace.

When all have drunk from the cup, place it back by the side of the fountain. Visualize your friends leaving the temple filled with light and love.

Start to become aware of your physical body and come out of this meditation as instructed on page 79.

Self-healing Meditation

This meditation can be used when you feel unwell, tired or when there is disharmony in your body, mind or spirit.

♦ Start your meditation by going to the temple described in the meditation for absent healing.

As you stand by the fountain, you are invited to enter it. Walking into the water, it feels warm upon your body. You feel it washing away all tiredness, disharmony or pain. As you look through the water towards the dome of the temple, the sun's rays make each droplet sparkle with its own rainbow. The beautiful coloured rainbows are absorbed into your body, mind and spirit as the water cascades upon you.

When you step out of the fountain, it feels as though you have cast off your old raiment and put on new. You feel full of life and vitality.

With gratitude and love, walk out of the temple and become aware of your physical body and the room where you are sitting. Slowly come out of this meditation as instructed on page 79.

The Crystal Chalice Meditation

This is a meditation for spiritual energy and can be used at the beginning of the day or before a healing session. Prepare yourself for this meditation by following the instructions given on pages 78–9.

♦ Imagine that you are sitting in a glass chalice. This chalice is bulb-shaped, wide at the bottom and narrow at the top, similar to a brandy glass. It is made in such a way that it reflects all the colours of the spectrum. As the light passes through the glass, the space between the chalice and your body is filled with red, orange, yellow, green, turquoise, blue, violet and magenta. These colours are constantly playing and dancing with each other. The chalice is strong and forms a protective web around you and, with its colours of ethereal light, represents your aura.

Looking up to the opening at the top of the chalice, you experience a shaft of white divine light flooding into your body through your crown chakra and radiating out into your aura. It fills you with energy and light. It fills you so that you are able to become a channel for healing, a channel of light and joy.

It continues to pour down until you are completely filled with light. It gives you energy, peace and joy.

When you are filled with this light, spend a few minutes in silence, thanking the spiritual world for this gift. Then return from this meditation as instructed on page 79.

The Chakra Meditation

Prepare yourself for this meditation by following the instructions given on pages 78–9.

♦ Bring your awareness into your spine, visualizing this as a beautiful column of golden light. Concentrate on the base of your spine, the coccyx. As you do this, you find yourself standing outside the base energy centre. Slowly walk inside. Entering, you find in front of you the bud of a red rose. Going up to this bud, place your hands around it and watch as it starts to open. When it has opened fully, walk into its centre and sit down. Becoming surrounded by the colour red, you are aware of its masculine energy. Your metabolic rate starts to increase and you are aware of the quickening of your heart beat. Your body temperature rises and you feel a sense of excitement. Instinctively you feel this colour grounding you to the planet earth. At the centre of this rose is an ascending shaft of white light. Standing up, walk into this light and let it gently lift you up into the second or sacral centre.

In this centre you see before you the bud of a deep orange chrysanthemum. Place your hands around this bud and watch it slowly open. Walking into its centre, sit down and feel the effect that the orange rays have upon your body. This colour mediates a much gentler energy, a feminine energy. Any depression that you may be experiencing is lifted and replaced by joy. In this colour you are able to lay down any tiredness and have your whole being re-energized. Looking to its centre, you see the white shaft of light. Get up and walk into it so that it may lift you up into the solar plexus centre.

Before you stands the bud of a daffodil. Go and place your hands around it. It responds to the warmth from your hands by opening. Walk into its centre and sit down. Becoming infused with the yellow ray, you feel yourself becoming detached from any problems that you are experiencing at this time or from any decisions that you have to make. In this detached state, you are able to see these problems more clearly and therefore see the correct solution to them. You become detached from family and friends and in so doing, you see that what they are doing and the path which they are treading is right for them. It is part of their learning and evolving. You know that you must watch them with love, always ready to help if they ask. Looking for the shaft of white light, get up and walk into it, allowing yourself to be lifted up into the heart centre.

At this centre you find the bud of a pale pink rose in the midst of a bed of green leaves. As you stand on these green leaves, any toxins in your body are eliminated and your positive and negative energies are brought into balance. You feel the three aspects of your being brought into harmony. Walking up to the pale pink bud, place your hands around it, allowing it to open in response to the warmth flowing from your hands. Walk into its centre and sit down, feeling the pale pink rays surround you and fill you with divine, spiritual love. This love is concentrated in your heart centre where it radiates out like the rays of the sun, falling upon those with whom you come into contact. Getting up and walking into the shaft of white light, you allow it to lift you up into the throat centre.

At this centre you stand before the bud of a cornflower. Placing your hands around it, the love from your heart centre flows down your arms and into your hands. Feeling the vibration of this love, the bud opens and invites you to sit at its centre. Surrounded by the blue rays, you feel all tension being released from your body and a sense of peace and deep relaxation pervading you. You instinctively know that this centre feels different from the others and you know that this is the bridge over which one must pass to transcend from the physical into the spiritual realm. If you feel that you are not yet ready to cross this bridge, you can stay wrapped in the mantle of peace and relaxation which this ray offers. If you wish to, and feel that it is right for you to cross, walk into the shaft of white light and allow it to lift you up into the brow centre.

This centre contains the bud of a deep indigo iris. As you gently touch it, it opens, inviting you to sit at its centre. As this deep indigo heightens your state of relaxation and peace, you feel able to come into contact with your higher self. In this state, you ask any questions which you are seeking answers to. It may be that you have come to a crossroads in your life and you are not sure which path to take. You may have problems or questions which you are seeking the answer to. In this silence, quietly ask and know that when the time is right, the answer will be given. This answer may come through another person, through a book which you pick up or through your intuition. When we work with this centre, the answers are sometimes given in picture form which pass before the inner eye. However we perceive the answer, rest assured, it will be given. Having asked and rested for a while in silence, peace and love, allow the shaft of white light which radiates from the centre of this flower to lift you up into the crown centre.

On entering this centre, you find yourself standing at the centre of a many-petalled lotus flower. The centre of this flower radiates a beautiful violet, giving to you the dignity and self-respect which you should have as a human being. As these violet rays radiate out, they change into a pale magenta which lifts up into the white light of God consciousness. Looking up into this light, the spiritual realm reveals to you all that you are ready to hear and see. As you raise your arms to embrace this light, a candle is placed into your hands. The flame of this candle represents your own spiritual awareness and truth. Take this flame and place it into your heart centre, letting its light be seen and shared by all those who are ready.

Thanking the spiritual realm for what you have been allowed to experience, you start to come back into earth consciousness. Using the cross of light within the circle of light, place it around each of the seven centres, starting with the crown and working down to the base. As you do this, watch as each flower closes. When you reach the base centre, feel the red which radiates here grounding you once more to the earth. When you are ready, open your eyes and be fully returned.

Evening Meditation

Prepare yourself for this meditation by following the instructions given on pages 78–9.

♦ It is evening, the last rays of the sun have sunk behind the hills, leaving the world wrapped in its dark cloak of night. The birds have returned to the trees; head beneath their wing, they dream of what the day has brought them. Domestic animals curl up in their baskets and in their kennels whilst farm animals bed down in their stalls. The night owl and other nocturnal creatures are the only souls about, on the prowl for food and sport.

The flowers have folded their petals, encasing within them the memory of the warmth and radiance of the sun. All is quiet and still.

In this stillness, reflect upon the day that has just passed, its triumphs, its mishaps, its sorrows and its joys. Take from it all that it has taught you and be thankful. Discard any negativity, anything that you no longer need, that should no longer be part of you.

Reflect upon your heart chakra. Enter this place which houses your higher or true self. Surrounded by the pale magenta light which is filling this space, allow it to enable you to let go of anything that you no longer need to keep and to fill the void which is left with pure spiritual love.

Allow this love to emanate out from your heart to fill the rest of your body. Extend it still further into the hearts of your family, friends and those you love. Ask that this love and peace may reach those places where there is war, strife, disharmony and tension.

Now place around your shoulders a beautiful blue cloak. Place its hood on your head and fasten it down the front. Visualize each of your centres of higher perception being closed and locked securely for the night. Wrapped in your mantle of peace and security, go to your bed and sleep so that your body may be re-energized in readiness for the dawn of another new day.

Good night

CHAPTER 7

Treating with Reflexology and Colour

On a patient's first visit, I always take down their particulars and medical history. This includes any drugs that they have taken or are taking, operations that they have undergone and illnesses that they have had. I then enquire about their current state of health and why they have come for treatment.

Time is then spent in talking to the person and encouraging them to talk to me, especially if I feel that the cause of their disease stems from an emotional or psychological problem. There are many people in the world who do not have a close friend in whom they can confide their innermost thoughts. It is so important to be able to express our feelings and problems. If we are unable to do this, they cause stress and tension which ultimately manifest as a physical ailment. Sometimes, we as therapists are used for this purpose. The person coming for treatment does not know us and therefore feels that they can confide in us that which they are unable to talk to anyone else about.

After I have listened to and talked to the patient, I explain to them the treatment procedure. I tell them that they can sleep, relax or talk to me during the treatment but that I need to know if they experience any pain. This initial treatment enables me to diagnose where there are blockages in the energy channels of the body. Having completed this, I then administer colour to the reflex zones which are related to the patient's complaint and into any zones which were painful. If an energy block has been present for some time, the zone which relates to it is sometimes too painful to touch. Using colour is a painless way of releasing the blockage without causing discomfort to the patient.

There are two ways in which colour can be administered to the reflex zones. The first is by allowing colour to flow through us into the patient. As I have already said, our physical body is the most perfect instrument which we have. If we learn to sensitize it, as described in the previous chapters, it can be used as a channel through which the healing colours of the universe flow. Before my day starts, I always light a candle and ask that I may be used as a channel. The flame of the candle for me represents the Christ light, but it can represent any deity or path that an individual is following. If you work with colour in this way, with dedication, do not be surprised if you sense a different colour from the one that you visualized being channelled through you. What we have to remember is that the higher powers know better than we do. I remember treating a patient with very advanced cancer. I visualized green and tried to bring it through my hands. Nothing happened. I then sensed a deep magenta being channelled through me. I watched this happening and asked why magenta and not green. The answer was given a few hours later when I picked up a book on healing in Atlantis. In this book, the question posed to one of the elders was whether red was used in healing. The answer given was yes, in some cases of cancer. Deep magenta is very close to red. When treating a patient, always tune in to your own intuition. Learn to listen and to trust it.

The second method of administration is through the reflexology crystal torch. This has already been described in the introduction. I invented and have been using this torch for about eight years with excellent results. It is ideal for people who find it difficult to visualize and channel colour, and for people who have had very little training in colour.

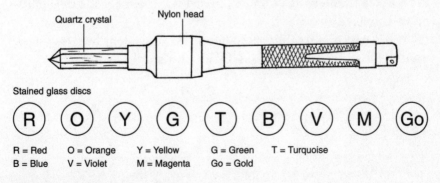

Fig. 28 The reflexology crystal torch

Charts have been included in this book showing the correct colours to use for various diseases. These are only guidelines. If your intuition tells you to use a different colour, then please do so. Whatever therapy we study, we always have to be given a firm foundation upon which to grow. Once we have built this foundation, then we have to grow from it by exploring and using our own ideas. These only come with experience.

After using a colour in the torch, shine the light from the torch through the crystal. This will cleanse the crystal of the colour's vibration, making it ready for the use of a new colour. At the end of each treatment, I ask that all negative energies in the crystal and stained glass be laid to the foundation by saying:

May the energies no longer required by this crystal be laid,
Earth to earth,
Water to water,
Fire to fire and
Air to air.

At the end of the day, I place the crystal into salt water for six hours in order to cleanse it thoroughly.

The length of time that a colour is channelled through the reflexes of the feet is approximately 60–90 seconds for each reflex. But having said this, remember that each person is an individual and therefore the time may differ with some people. Again, learn to listen to your intuition.

At the end of each treatment, use the torch to balance the chakras on the spinal reflex. Do this by bringing the feet together and placing the torch between the feet on each individual chakra, using the appropriate colour.

At the end of a treatment, I always ask the patient how they feel, what they have experienced and if they wish to ask any questions.

The Attributes of Each Colour

Red

Red is the colour which has the slowest wave lengths. It is at the heat end of the spectrum and represents fire.

Red is the symbol of life, strength and vitality. In the aura a clear bright red shows generosity, ambition and affection. An excess of red in the aura means strong physical propensities. Dark red indicates deep passion, love, courage, hatred, anger, etc. The dark cloudy shades of a colour are always negative. Reddish-brown shows sensuality and voluptuousness and cloudy red greed and cruelty. Crimson indicates lower passions and desires, and scarlet lust.

Red is the dominant colour of the base chakra and is the colour which earths us to this planet. Children tend to love this colour because, until they reach puberty, they are not fully earthed.

Ronald Hunt, in his book *The Seven Keys to Colour Healing*, calls this ray the great energizer, the father of vitality. According to him, red splits the ferric salt crystals into iron and salt. The red corpuscles in the blood absorb the iron and the salt is eliminated by the kidneys and the skin. This makes it a good colour with which to treat anaemia or iron deficiency.

Red is a very powerful energizer and stimulant and I feel that it is related to the masculine energy. Through its effect on the haemoglobin, it increases energy, raises body temperature and improves the circulation. It is therefore a good colour to use for paralysis.

Because it is a powerful stimulant and energizer, red is not used a great deal in therapy, especially if there are anxiety or emotional disturbances. The exception to this is in the base chakra. Here it is used to clear blockages and to bring this energy centre back into balance.

When used in conjunction with its complementary colour of turquoise, it is beneficial for infections. The red increases the blood circulation, enabling it to cope more adequately with the infection, whilst the turquoise helps to reduce any inflammation. In reflexology, these two colours are used on the reflex zones related to any part of the body where there is inflammation.

Contra-indications for Red

Red should not be used on people suffering from asthma, high blood pressure, heart disease or epilepsy. Orange should be used where red has been indicated.

The use of red in treatment

Reflex	Complaint	Colour	Complementary
Lungs	Pneumonia	Red	Turquoise
Colon	Constipation	Red	Turquoise
Uterus	Infertility	Red	Turquoise
Ovaries	Infertility	Red	Turquoise
Base chakra	Imbalance	Red	—

Two Meditations with Red

Before starting these meditations, read the instructions given for meditation on pages 78–9.

♦ *Meditation 1*

When your body is relaxed and comfortable and your mind still and quiet, imagine that you are sitting in the countryside. It is a warm summer's evening and the sun is just beginning to set. As it starts to sink below the horizon, the sky becomes ablaze with colour. It is filled with all the shades and hues of red which gradually fade into a pale pink. The colours are alive and dancing. They speak to you as they surround your physical body. Try to sense how this colour is affecting you, physically, mentally and spiritually, as it is absorbed into your body. Stay with this image for as long as you feel is right for you.

Now that the sun has set and darkness fallen, everything has become very still and silent. Listen to this silence and try to reflect upon yourself and your experiences during this meditation.

When you are ready, gradually start to increase your inhalation and exhalation, becoming aware of the room in which you are sitting. In your own time, open your eyes and be fully returned to earth consciousness.

♦ Meditation 2

It is a cold winter's evening and the world is wrapped in her dark mantle of night. The sky is clear and there is frost on the ground.

As you approach the front door of your home, you look up into the clear sky, seeing it filled with twinkling jewels of light set against a deep indigo background. Your hands and feet feel cold, even though they are protected with warm clothing, and your face, which is just visible above your thick winter's coat, feels numb.

You open your front door with relief, enter your home and remove your outdoor clothing. Walking into the sitting room, you enter the glow being created by the log fire which burns in the grate. As you sit down on the hearth rug by the fire, you feel its warmth penetrating your chilled body. Looking into the fire you watch the flames dancing and creating smoke which swirls and winds its way up the chimney. The colours in the flames range from the deepest to the palest red, intermingled with orange, white and occasionally blue.

As you concentrate upon these flames you feel them inviting you to become one of them. You accept and in so doing they allow you to feel the warm, deeply energizing and earthing colour of red. As you dance and play with them, you become aware of the presence of other beings. Could it be the salamanders, those elementals responsible for fire? Ask them to communicate with you and then sit in silence, listening intuitively for them to respond.

Are they asking you to take the flame that you are experiencing into your heart so that you can take it out into the world where mankind can benefit from its warmth, light and joy, taking it especially to those places where there is darkness and emptiness? Listen carefully and answer as you feel is right for you.

Returning from this meditation and becoming aware of your physical body, if you feel that it is right for you, take the flame that you became into your heart. Take it out into the world so that those who are ready may share your experiences with you.

Orange

Orange is the symbol of energy. In the aura, a bright clear orange denotes health and vitality, a deep orange, pride, and a muddy cloudy orange, a low intellect. An excess of orange in the aura shows an abundance of vital dynamic force.

Orange is the dominant colour of the sacral chakra and is related to the female reproductive organs and the adrenal glands. It is akin to the feminine energy, the energy of creation. It is more gentle than the dynamic, masculine energy of red but is complementary to it. Therefore these two colours should be worked in balance and harmony. Orange is the colour of joy and dance.

This colour is also associated with the splenic chakra. It is through this chakra that prana or etheric energy is absorbed, split up into the individual colours of the spectrum and distributed to the relevant chakra. Orange is therefore a good colour to use for fatigue and exhaustion.

The orange ray is used to treat kidney stones and stones in the gall bladder. Frequently these stones are caused by our own bitterness and resentment against other people or life in general. Orange has proved beneficial in cases of chronic bronchitis and with regular treatment can clear any build-up of phlegm and the cough which accompanies it. Orange has an antispasmodic effect and should therefore be used for muscle spasms and cramp.

Meditation with Orange

Prepare yourself for meditation by following the instructions given on pages 78–9.

For this meditation, you will need a bowl containing five or six oranges and a knife.

♦ Sit in a place where you can clearly see the oranges and start your meditation by just looking at them. Observe how they have been placed in the bowl. Are they all the same size? Is their colour uniform or does the colour vary? Are they emitting an aroma? Is the texture of the skin the same for each orange, or does it differ?

After contemplating the bowl of oranges for about ten minutes, take one of them into your hands. Carefully look for any variation in the colour or texture of the skin. Now cut it open and compare the difference in colour between the flesh and the skin. Place one half of the orange onto the palm of your left hand and place the palm of your right hand about 2 inches above it. Close your eyes and try to feel the vibration of this colour through the chakra in the palm of your right hand. Breathe in the aroma and see if it provokes any memories of past events which you may have forgotten. Look at any memories or pictures which may come into your mind. When you feel that you have experienced all that you are able to, place the orange back into the bowl.

Sit quietly and try to tune into your own body. Try to feel the sacral chakra which is situated just below the umbilical scar. Gently start to breathe in orange, bringing it from the earth and into this centre. As you exhale, allow the orange colour to radiate out into your aura. Feel yourself becoming energized and filled with joy. Allow any depression that you may have been experiencing to be dissolved.

When you are ready, end this meditation by gradually increasing your inhalation and exhalation and feeling yourself being returned to everyday consciousness.

The Use of Orange in Treatment

Reflex	Complaint	Colour	Complementary
Lungs	Bronchitis	Orange	Blue
Head	Head colds	Orange	Blue
Thyroid	Under-active	Orange	Blue
Gall Bladder	Stones	Orange	Blue
Kidneys	Stones	Orange	Blue
Small intestine	General treatment	Orange	Gold
Ovaries	Benign cysts	Orange	Blue
Uterus	Prolapse and fibroids	Orange	Blue
Prostate	General treatment	Orange	Blue
Sacral chakra	Imbalance	Orange	Blue
Spleenic chakra	Fatigue	Orange	Blue

Gold

Gold comprises yellow and orange and is the complementary colour of indigo. It is the colour of wisdom, associated with mysticism. This is portrayed in the gold halos shown around the heads of saints. In the colour gold, the yellow, pertaining to the intellect, has been transmuted to the wisdom of Cosmic consciousness, which, when realized, is accepted with an all-knowing sense of joy and bliss.

Gold has the healing quality associated with vitality. It is therefore used, with its complementary indigo, down the spinal column to revitalize the nervous system. Applied to the spleen, gold has a reaction similar to that of orange. It gives vitality to the human system and has a beneficial effect on the skeletal system.

The Use of Gold in Treatment

Reflex	Complaint	Colour	Complementary
Spine	Revitalize	Gold	Indigo
Spleen	Revitalize	Orange	Blue

Meditation Using Both Indigo and Gold

Prepare yourself for meditation by following the instructions on pages 78–9.

♦ The hot rays of the summer sun have sunk beneath the horizon, heralding the darkness and silence of night. With the rays of light vanquished, the sky takes on the deep indigo of night. The only part of the sky not vibrating to this colour is the circular halo, comprising yellow, gold and orange, surrounding the almost full moon. On such a clear night, the light from the stars take on a vibrant golden hue.

Imagine yourself to be part of this scenario. Allow the deep indigo of the night to gently fold round and cloak your human form. In so doing, tension and stress which has accumulated during the day is slowly released. Feel the penetrating rays of this colour ease any pain that you may be suffering.

As your body relaxes and allows the strong sense of peace and stillness to pervade it, visualize the golden shafts of light from the stars entering the top of your head, travelling through your skull and down your spinal column. This promotes a tingling sensation as your nervous system is re-energized.

Remain with this visualization for as long as you feel comfortable. If you drift into sleep, don't worry, the body needs to do this. When you feel ready to come out of the visualization, start to increase your inhalation and exhalation. Envisage each of your chakras closing, like a flower returning to a bud. Gently open your eyes and feel yourself returned to everyday awareness.

Yellow

Yellow is the symbol of the mind and intellect and is the dominant colour of the solar plexus chakra. This energy centre controls the digestive system and helps to purify the body through its eliminating action on the liver and intestines.

In the aura, golden yellow denotes high soul qualities, a pale primrose yellow, great intellectual power, a dark dingy yellow, jealousy and suspicion, and a dull, lifeless yellow, false optimism. An excess of yellow in the aura shows an abundance of mental power.

The yellow rays carry positive magnetic currents which are inspiring and stimulating. They strengthen the nerves and stimulate the higher mentality. This is the colour which activates the motor nerves in the physical body and can therefore generate energy in the muscles. If any part of the body lacks the energy of this colour, it can manifest as partial or complete paralysis. It is therefore a colour which is used to treat these conditions.

Yellow works with the skin by improving its texture, cleansing and healing scars and other disorders such as eczema. It is used for all rheumatic and arthritic conditions because it helps to break down the calcium deposits which have formed in the joints.

Yellow is the colour of detachment and if used in excess, a person can become detached from people and the environment.

Two Meditations with Yellow

Before starting these meditations, read the instructions given on pages 78–9.

♦ *Meditation 1*

It is a warm summer's day and you are lying on a golden sandy beach in a small cove. You are alone. The only sounds to be heard are the waves of the sea as they break on the shore and the cry of seagulls overhead. As you lie on the sand bathed in the warmth of the sun, a gentle breeze plays upon your body. Surrounding the cove are grey cliffs which have green rock plants growing out of their crevices. The sky above is a pale blue and has tiny clouds sailing across it with the breeze. The atmosphere is filled with peace and tranquillity.

Closing your eyes and releasing any thoughts from your mind, bring your concentration into your physical body. Feel it surrounded by the golden yellow rays which are radiating from the sand and the sun.

Slowly, you feel yourself becoming detached from the world and its problems. In this state, you are able to look objectively at any of your own problems to which you are trying to find a solution. You are able to look, with love, at family and friends and to realize that what they are doing is right for them and that through their actions they are learning, growing and evolving. You understand that you cannot possess or judge them or anyone else with whom you come into contact. Lying quietly, ask to be shown the correct solution to any problems that you have or, if you have reached a crossroads in your life, ask to be shown the correct path to take. At times, the path which we are shown is difficult and uninviting, full of hurdles and difficult decisions. We have been given free will and can choose to forgo this path for an easier one. If we do this, eventually we will again be confronted with the original path because it is only by taking this road that we are able to evolve.

Place the palms of your hands upon the sand. Feel the tiny grains trickle over and through your fingers. Through the chakras in the palms of your hands, try to feel the vibration of this colour. Now visualize a shaft of pure yellow light entering through the soles of your feet, into your solar plexus. See your solar plexus become a golden living disc of light. As you exhale, allow this colour to radiate out into your aura.

When you are ready, start to increase your inhalation and exhalation, gradually returning to earth consciousness. Close down your chakras as described on page 79.

◆ *Meditation 2*

Visualize a sunflower growing in a garden. In your visualization take particular notice of the flower, how large it is and how many petals it has. Look inside the petals to its centre where the deep golden stamens of the plant grow.

Sitting quietly, take this golden yellow flower into your solar plexus. Allow its petals to become rays of translucent light which penetrate the organs and muscles situated in this part of your body. From the flower's centre, watch as a shaft of yellow light rays out into your aura.

In silence, try to experience how this colour affects you mentally, physically and spiritually. Take this colour in your visualization to any other part of your body where you feel that it would be beneficial.

When you are ready, start to increase your inhalation and exhalation. Become aware of the room or place where you are sitting. Now open your eyes.

The Use of Yellow in Treatment

Reflex	*Complaint*	*Colour*	*Complementary*
Spine	Paralysis	Yellow	Violet
Parathyroids	Osteoporosis	Yellow	Violet
Shoulder	Frozen shoulder	Yellow	Violet
Stomach	Indigestion	Yellow	Violet
Pancreas	Diabetes	Yellow	Violet
Sacroiliac joint	Arthritis	Yellow	Violet
Anus	Piles	Yellow	Violet
Solar plexus chakra	General treatment	Yellow	Orange

Green

Green is the midway colour in the spectrum, being neither at the hot nor the cold end. It is the colour of balance, harmony and sympathy and is the dominant colour of the heart chakra.

In the aura, bright, clear greens symbolize good qualities; light greens, prosperity and success; mid green, adaptability and versatility; clear green, sympathy; dark green, deceit; and olive green, treachery and double nature in a person. An excess of green in the aura denotes individualism and independence.

Green has antiseptic properties enabling it to be used for infections. It can detoxify the body and bring the negative and positive energies into balance. It also balances the body, mind and spirit. When these three aspects of a person are brought into balance, it creates wholeness.

Green will cleanse the etheric body when administered through the throat chakra. Being the dominant colour of the heart chakra, it can also be used to treat certain heart disorders. If the disorder stems from an emotional origin, rose pink and pale violet should be used instead.

The Use of Green in Treatment

Reflex	Complaint	Colour	Complementary
Colon	Toxicity	Green	Magenta
Liver	Toxicity	Yellow	Orange
Kidneys	Toxicity	Green	Magenta
Heart	Balance	Green	Magenta
Throat chakra	Cleanse etheric body	Green	Magenta
Heart chakra	Balance	Green	Magenta

Meditation with Green

Before starting this meditation, read the instructions given on pages 78–9.

♦ When you have relaxed and made your body comfortable, imagine that you are walking through a forest. The path upon which you walk is carpeted with fallen leaves and twigs in various stages of decay.

The roots of the trees which protrude above the earth make their own intricate design. The trees tower majestically above you, stretching up their branches towards the light of the heavens. The air feels damp through lack of prolonged sunshine and the only noise is the sound of the crackling twigs and rustling leaves which come into contact with your feet as you walk along. All else is silent. Looking up towards the sky, you can see how the branches and leaves intertwine with each other, designing and creating archways throughout the forest. These only allow very thin shafts of light to penetrate through.

Finding a dry piece of ground beneath one of the trees, sit down with your back against the tree, breathing in the atmosphere and silence. Talk to the tree and ask it to share its energy with you. Feel that energy entering your body, travelling through your spine and energizing the nerves, organs and cells. Thank the tree.

Lie down beneath the tree and look up at its branches. These are filled with leaves displaying the various shades of green. Where the light filters through, the leaves take on a lighter colour than those in the shade. Try to sense and feel with your body the various shades of this colour. Take note of your experiences and try to ascertain which shade of green you have the greatest affinity with.

As you inhale, visualize a shaft of this colour horizontally entering your heart chakra, removing any blockages which may be present. As you exhale, allow the colour to radiate out into your aura. Try to be aware of this colour bringing the positive and negative energies of your body into balance. Also of bringing your body, mind and spirit into harmony.

Now breathe this colour into your throat chakra. Visualize it freeing the energy channels in the etheric body of any toxins or blockages.

When you feel ready, relax for five to ten minutes, observing any changes which may have taken place within you.

Start to increase your inhalation and exhalation and close this meditation as described on page 79.

Turquoise

Turquoise is the last colour which appears out of the blue half of the spectrum. It is a colour which is not normally associated with the seven main chakras.

In eastern esoteric teaching, the heart chakra, which radiates green, is always connected with the thymus gland. This is a gland which, according to the medical profession, atrophies after puberty. Before that, it functions as part of the immune system. The thymus has its own minor chakra which is one of the twenty-one minor chakras in the physical body. Through the practice of yoga and meditation, I have come to realize that as we enter the Aquarian Age, this minor chakra is enlarging into the eighth major chakra. I feel that it is the chakra which will be responsible for raising us into the higher level of consciousness of the New Age. Not only do we as human beings have to achieve this but also the whole of the planet. We can either help the earth in this task or let it be destroyed.

When the thymus chakra starts to open and expand, it encompasses the heart and throat chakra, plus many of the smaller centres situated in the throat, chest, shoulders and hands. I feel that those who have reached this level of development have the responsibility of trying to help their fellow human beings, who as yet do not understand, also to evolve into the New Age.

Turquoise, being associated with the thymus chakra, is a colour which works with the immune system and is used to boost this system. This could be a good colour for people suffering with Aids, helping to prolong their life by strengthening the immune system which the Aids virus destroys. Turquoise can also be used where inflammation is present. For this, it is particularly beneficial when used with its complementary colour red. Red brings a greater supply of blood to the area of inflammation, destroying any bacteria that are present, whilst turquoise helps to soothe and bring down the inflammation. If a person is suffering from a bacterial or virus infection or has just recovered from one, the lymph reflexes should be treated with this colour.

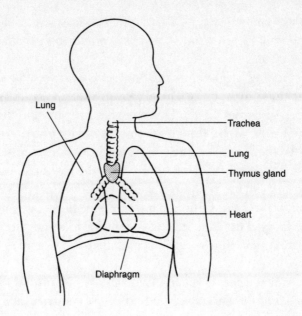

Fig. 29 The position of the thymus

The Use of Turquoise in Treatment

Reflex	Complaint	Colour	Complementary
Throat	Sore throat	Turquoise	Red
Ear	Infections	Turquoise	Red
Kidneys	Nephritis	Turquoise	Red
Bladder	Cystitis	Turquoise	Red
Lymphatic system	General treatment	Turquoise	Red
Thymus gland	General treatment	Turquoise	Red

Meditation with turquoise

Prepare yourself for meditation by following the instructions given on pages 78–9.

♦ In your imagination, take yourself to a place where you are surrounded by mountains, their peaks soaring up towards the heavens. On the summit of the tallest of these is snow which, due to the cold climate of that altitude, remains throughout the year. The whiteness of the snow glistens and looks radiant in the light of the sun.

Finding a gentle, undulating path, start to walk along it and up into these mountains. The landscape that you see varies from sheer-faced grey rock to gently sloping land, covered in grass and mountain plants. Upon this green pasture, sheep graze.

Walking on, you hear the sound of water and you see to your right a tiny waterfall cascading down the rocks and boulders. Where the sun catches the water, rainbows appear, creating living, dancing bands of colour. Continuing past the waterfall, you notice in one of the faces of the mountain what appears to be an entrance. On investigation, you find yourself standing at the entrance to a cave. You walk in.

At first it seems very dark and airless. As your eyes become accustomed to the darkness, you find yourself surrounded by stalagmites and stalactites but when you look at the floor of the cave, you find that it is covered with turquoise stones of all shapes and sizes.

Finding a ledge in the rock, sit down and pick up some of these pieces of turquoise. Look at their colour and for any variation in this colour. Place a piece onto the palm of your left hand, then place the palm of your right hand about 1½ inches above it. Try to feel for any vibrations or sensations that it transmits. Now place this stone upon any part of your physical body where you feel that it would be beneficial. Feel its vibration bringing you back into harmony and balance. Feel it strengthening and energizing your immune system. Lastly, place it over your thymus gland. Concentrate on this gland and visualize your piece of turquoise activating the chakra in it.

Sit very quietly. Visualize yourself surrounded by the energies which are being emitted from these stones which lie on the ground. Feel their energies entering your body through the chakras on the soles of your feet. Reflect on any changes which may take place within you, physically, mentally and emotionally.

When you are ready, end this meditation by gently increasing your inhalation and exhalation, closing down your chakras and returning to everyday consciousness.

Blue

Blue is the dominant colour of the throat chakra and lies at the cold end of the spectrum. It symbolizes inspiration, devotion, peace and tranquillity. This makes it an excellent colour to use with meditation and in places of healing.

In the aura, a deep clear blue shows pure religious feeling, a pale ethereal blue, devotion to a noble ideal, and bright blue, loyalty and sincerity. An excess of blue in the aura signifies an artistic, harmonious nature and spiritual understanding.

This colour can be used as a protection. To do this, visualize yourself putting on a long blue cloak which reaches down to your feet, with a hood which you place over your head. Fasten the cloak with its full-length zip. As you fasten your cloak, so you protect yourself from any outside influence or negative energies. You allow to enter only what you choose.

In the New Testament, the Virgin Mary is depicted as wearing a mantle of blue. Many of the masters, those who have reached a state of spiritual enlightenment, have interpreted this as being an abundance of blue in her aura, denoting spirituality, devotion and protection.

Unlike red, blue is a colour which slows down and expands. A room painted in this colour will appear to be much larger. It is used to treat tension, fear, palpitations and insomnia. A person suffering with insomnia can help themselves by sleeping in blue sheets with either white or blue night clothes. A low wattage blue light bulb can also be used, all night if necessary.

Blue will reduce inflammation and can be administered to the relevant reflexes on the hands or feet. Because it is the dominant colour of the throat chakra, it is frequently used for problems occurring in this area, for example, laryngitis, sore throat, tonsilitis and goitres.

When blue is administered with its complementary colour orange, it brings about a state of peaceful joy.

Meditation with Blue

Prepare yourself for meditation by following the instructions on pages 78–9.

◆ It is a clear, pleasantly warm day in spring and you are walking through a wood carpeted with bluebells. Finding a fallen tree trunk, sit down and look at this spectacle of colour and splendour. Observing these flowers, notice how wonderfully and intricately they are made. Each tiny bell possesses its own individuality of colour and shape.

Closing your eyes and visualizing one of these flowers, you find that the bell shape of the flower starts to expand, until it completely surrounds you and you find yourself sitting inside it. The stamens provide a pillow upon which to rest your head. Lie back and feel the softness of the petals encircling you like a soft mantle. The blue rays emanating from the petals play upon your body, releasing tension in your muscles and organs. Your inhalation and exhalation deepens as your body relaxes. As you inhale, you breathe this colour into your body through all the pores of your skin. If there is any pain or inflammation in your body, visualize this colour surrounding the affected part, bringing relaxation and healing.

You are beginning to feel a deep sense of peace and tranquillity. You lose sense of time and place and you start to become part of the peace which surrounds you. Your physical body melts into this atmosphere of tranquillity and you begin to sense your higher self. You become conscious that it is inviting you to lay before it any problems or worries that you may have. Sitting in silence and doing this, you intuitively know that when the time is right, the answers to these problems will be given. Sometimes they are given through a friend or through a book that we are reading. At other times they come through our own intuition. We have to learn to wait and to have trust.

At the end of your time of silence, feel yourself being filled with that peace and tranquillity which passeth all man's understanding. As you slowly start to increase your inhalation and exhalation, the flower of the bluebell starts to shrink and you become aware of your body sitting in the place which you chose for this meditation. Coming back into earth consciousness, end this meditation by closing down your centres of higher perception.

The Use of Blue in Treatment

Reflex	Complaint	Colour	Complementary
Head	Epilepsy	Blue	Orange
Neck	Stiff neck	Blue	Orange
Eyes	Glaucoma	Blue	Orange
Thyroid	Goitre and over-active	Blue	Orange
Lungs	Asthma and pleurisy	Blue	Orange
Heart	Tachycardia and palpitations	Blue	Orange
Solar plexus	Tension and stress	Blue	Orange
Liver	Jaundice	Blue	Orange
Stomach	Ulcers	Blue	Orange
Ileo-caecal valve	Constipation	Blue	Orange
Colon	Diarrhoea	Blue	Orange
Ovaries	During pregnancy	Blue	Orange
Uterus	During pregnancy	Blue	Orange
Breast	Mastitis	Blue	Orange
Prostate	Enlarged	Blue	Orange

Indigo

The colour indigo comprises blue and violet and is the dominant colour of the brow chakra. It works with the pituitary gland and encompasses the organs of sight and hearing. It also embraces other aspects of the face.

Combining both the blue and violet ray, it speaks of deep devotion, carried with a sense of dignity and unconditional love. It is also responsible for transcendent vision and for allowing us the ability to hear the voice of our own intuition.

Indigo, found at the cool end of the spectrum, is a ray which is cooling and astringent. It has the capacity to induce anaesthesia in the physical body, this makes it a powerful painkiller. It is a colour which helps to purify the bloodstream and the psychic currents found in the aura. It is also a colour which is very helpful for nosebleeds.

Owing to its connection to the organs of sight and hearing, it is a colour used to treat cataracts and deafness. If suffering from either of these complaints, we have to look at the cause of the physical disease. Any problem relating to the eye can be caused by our unwillingness to see things that are beneficial for us, and also by our refusing to see someone else's point of view. This attitude could lead to a persecution complex, making our outlook on life warped.

Deafness can be caused by an accident or severe shock, but it can also be the result of our unwillingness to hear things that may be for our own good. In such a case, we are giving our subconscious a silent command to shut our ears.

The Use of Indigo in Treatment

Reflex	*Complaint*	*Colour*	*Complementary*
Head	Headaches, neuralgic pain and insomnia	Indigo	Gold
Spine	Pain	Indigo	Gold
Sinuses	Pain from sinusitis, colds and catarrh	Indigo	Gold
Eyes	Cataracts and eye strain	Indigo	Gold
Ears	Deafness	Indigo	Gold
Heart	Angina	Indigo	Gold
Shoulder	Muscular strains or tension	Indigo	Gold
Liver	Hepatitis	Indigo	Gold
Small intestine	Inflammation	Indigo	Gold
Sciatic loop	Sciatica	Indigo	Gold

Meditation with Indigo

See *Meditation using both indigo and gold*

Violet

Violet is the colour of spirituality, self-respect and dignity, a colour frequently needed by people who have no respect for their thoughts, feelings or physical body. These people can love others but are unable to love themselves. When I sense this in a patient, I tell them to look in a mirror first thing in the morning and last thing at night and to tell the image that they see how much they love it. Patients frequently laugh at this advice. They feel self-conscious when they start to practise it, but are amazed at how effective it can be.

Violet is the colour related to insight and the higher self. It is an inspirational colour. Many musicians, poets and painters have written that their moments of greatest inspiration came when they were surrounded by the violet ray.

Violet is the dominant colour of the crown chakra. In the aura, a deep purple denotes high spiritual attainment and holy love. It proclaims the divine radiance. A pale lilac shows cosmic consciousness and love for humanity, a bluish purple, transcendent idealism.

This is a very beneficial colour for psychological disorders such as schizophrenia and manic depression. It also helps sciatica, diseases of the scalp and all disorders connected with the nervous system.

The Use of Violet in Treatment

Reflex	Complaint	Colour	Complementary
Head	Scalp complaints – baldness	Violet	Yellow
Spine	Spinal meningitis	Violet	Yellow
Heart	Broken heart (emotional)	Violet/rose pink	

Meditation with Violet

Prepare yourself for meditation by following the instructions given on pages 78–9.

♦ It is a warm and sunny autumn day. You are standing outside a small church, situated in the countryside. It is surrounded by fields in which animals graze. The leaves on the trees have turned into their autumnal colours of yellow, orange, red and brown. Some of them have already fallen, making a rich and varied coloured carpet upon the earth. Birds sing overhead and there is a distant hum of passing traffic.

Walk up to the door of the church. Push it open and walk inside. Here the air smells musty and feels cool in comparison to the warmth of the sun outside. Standing and listening, you become aware of the still and silent atmosphere. Allow this atmosphere to enter every cell of your being, slowing down your respiration and giving you a feeling of peace and relaxation.

As your eyes become accustomed to the comparative darkness, you notice the statues of the angels and saints which are standing around the church. In the far left-hand corner stands a statue of the Virgin Mary carrying the Christ child. Look up the aisle towards the sanctuary and you will see the altar decked in white linen, edged with a deep layer of lace. Upon it stands a crucifix and six candles. A small sanctuary light burns above it. The church is surrounded by beautiful stained glass windows, depicting events in the life of Christ. As the sun shines through these windows, shafts of pure violet light stream into the church.

Walk to one of the pews and sit down in these shafts of violet light. Close your eyes and feel yourself immersed in this colour. Feel your aura and every cell in your body absorbing its vibration. It gives to you the feeling of dignity and self-respect that each one of us should have as human beings, dignity and respect for your feelings, thoughts and body. With these feelings, you are raised to a higher level of consciousness where you are allowed to glimpse your true self, the eternal part of you which has no beginning and no ending. You are shown that this is the real you and that your physical body is the sacred instrument in which you live on the earth plane. You begin to see what a very beautiful instrument the physical body is, capable of self-healing when given the right conditions. You are also told that all human life is sacred and, as a healer, you must respect this and allow your own instrument to be used as a channel for the flow of the healing power of the universe. Sit for a while and reflect on these thoughts.

When you feel ready, stand and walk towards the door. Look around the church once more and thank the angels, saints and your higher self for the experience that you have been given.

Walking out of the church, start to increase your inhalation and exhalation, uniting yourself with your physical body. End this meditation in the normal way

Magenta

Situated above the crown chakra are three higher chakras. These can be experienced through deep meditation.

The first of these radiates a pale magenta light, the second, the white light of God consciousness, and the third radiates that sacred darkness out of which all things become manifest.

Magenta is the colour of letting go. In order to experience these three higher chakras we have first to let go of our thoughts and emotions. We are then able to rise in consciousness to the magenta above the crown chakra. Here, we have to let go of our physical body in order to raise our consciousness into the white light of God consciousness and then into the sacred darkness.

On a physical mental level, magenta enables us to let go of ideas and thought patterns which are no longer right for us. If we hold on to ideas and conditioning which originated in our childhood or adolescence, we become fixed and rigid and this prevents us from growing and evolving. To let go is sometimes difficult because it involves change and this can cause insecurity and uncertainty. If we are able to see these changes as a challenge, then they enable us to move forward.

In letting go and flowing with the energies of life, we no longer have a set routine or pattern. This can be very unsettling for our personality but for our spirit it is bliss because it can move unhindered towards the vision which it had before it incarnated into a physical body. Once we have entered into a physical body the vision is lost to our normal senses but the spirit remembers and will pursue it at all costs.

On the emotional level, magenta signifies letting go of feelings which are no longer relevant. Perhaps we are still living in a relationship that has ended or in a situation that has passed. In order to grow and learn from our present situation, we have to let go emotionally of the past. Again, not easy.

On the physical level, it means relinquishing a physical activity which is no longer right for us. It could be a sport or some other activity in which we are partaking.

When magenta turns into a very pale pink, it becomes the colour of spiritual love. If a person is suffering from a 'broken heart', this colour can be applied to the heart chakra to heal and to replace the emptiness frequently experienced with spiritual love. If I am treating a person who is experiencing the loss of a dear one or the ending of a relationship, I tell them that I have planted a pale pink rose, which is still in bud, in their heart chakra. I tell them to water the rose every day through concentration and meditation, until it comes into full bloom.

Magenta comprises red and violet. Red, on the electromagnetic spectrum, follows infra-red which is a burning ray, and violet comes just below ultraviolet which is also a burning ray. For this reason mag-enta is used to treat malignant tumours.

May I suggest that if you, the reader, choose to work with reflexology and colour, you also learn to tune into your higher self in order that the correct colour may be channelled. Always remember, none of us are healers, only channels through which colour and the healing power of the universe can flow.

The Use of Magenta in Treatment

Reflex	Complaint	Colour	Complementary
Pituitary gland	Tumours	Magenta	Green
Eyes	Detached retina	Magenta	Green
Ears	Tinnitus	Magenta	Green
Lungs	Cancer	Magenta	Green
Heart	Thrombosis	Magenta	Green
Stomach	Cancer	Magenta	Green
Kidneys	Nephroma	Magenta	Green
	Water retention		
Small intestine	Cancer	Magenta	Green
Colon	Cancer	Magenta	Green
Uterus	Uterine cancer	Magenta	Green
Breast	Cysts	Magenta	Green
	Cancer	Magenta	Green
Testes	Malignant tumour	Magenta	Green

Meditation with Magenta

Prepare yourself for meditation by following the instructions given on pages 78–9.

♦ Picture before your inner eye a golden circle. Inside this circle is a beautiful magnolia flower in full bloom. Its petals are white with stripes of magenta running through them. These stripes are very narrow at the base of the petal, gradually widening until they join at the top of the flower, encircling it in a band of pale magenta light.

As you concentrate on this flower, visualize it growing bigger until its petals enfold you and you are sitting at its centre.

Sit still for a moment and try to feel the softness of the petals that are surrounding you. Be aware of the soft glow of magenta light that radiates from this flower and is absorbed by every cell in your physical body. Sitting in this colour, allow yourself to let go of any tension or pain, any emotional or mental problems that may be upsetting you. Let go of anything that you feel is no longer right for you. This could be a relationship, conditioning or an old habit. It is only by letting go of these things, no matter how painful, that we are able to grow and evolve. If you are at a crossroads in your life, let go of it. By doing this, we can frequently see the path that we are meant to take more clearly.

Having laid aside all the things that you no longer need, look up to the top of the flower. See how the magenta shines from the top of the petals and lifts up into the white light of God consciousness, the white light which was born out of the sacred darkness and which contains all things. Allow yourself to be gently drawn up into this light and there absorb the peace, understanding and reality which it can give.

After a while, into your hands is placed a lighted candle. The flame of this candle represents all that this white light has revealed to you. Take the flame and place it in your heart chakra where it burns as a symbol of the divine spark which is in each one of us.

Having done this, slowly start to return to earth consciousness by descending out of the white light into the magenta. Allow the petals of this flower to get smaller until you are again sitting outside it and it becomes a picture before your inner eye. Increase your inhalation and exhalation and start to become aware of your physical body. When you feel ready, open your eyes and be fully returned to earth consciousness. Now close down your centres of higher perception as normal.

Meditation with Pale Pink

Prepare yourself for meditation by following the instructions given on pages 78–9.

♦ Bring your concentration into your heart centre. Visualize this as a small chamber that you are about to enter.

Inside, you find growing a pale pink rose which is still in bud. Go up to that bud and place your hands around it, allowing warmth and love from your higher self to flow through your hands and into the flower.

Watch as it slowly starts to open, revealing to you the delicacy with which each petal is fashioned, the subtle intonation of the colour, from pale pink to a deep rich pink at the outer edges and base of each petal.

Contemplating this flower, you feel it radiating to you a sense of deep spiritual love, the love that is permanent and unchanging. This love starts to fill your heart chakra and any emptiness that you are feeling within yourself. Every aspect of your being is touched by these rays of love. Sit for a while in silence and reflect upon this.

When you are ready, gently start to increase your inhalation and exhalation and become united with your physical body. Look into your heart chakra and see that flower, in full bloom, still radiating its love to you. Remember to care for it each day in your meditation.

Colour Guidelines for Reflexology

Reflex	General reflex colour	Complaint	Colours for specific complaints	
			Treatment colour	Complementary colour
Spine	Gold	Paralysis	Yellow	Violet
		Spinal meningitis	Violet	Yellow
		Pain	Indigo	Gold
Head	Blue	Epilepsy	Blue	Orange
		Headaches; neuralgic pain	Indigo	Gold
		Insomnia	Indigo	Gold
		Head colds	Orange	Blue
		Scalp complaints	Violet	Yellow
Pituitary	Indigo	Tumours	Magenta	Green
Sinuses	Indigo	Sinusitis, colds and catarrh	Indigo	Gold
		To reduce pain	Indigo	Gold
Neck	Blue	Stiff neck	Blue	Orange
		Sore throat	Turquoise	Red
Eyes	Indigo	Eye strain	Indigo	Gold
		Cataracts	Indigo	Gold
		Glaucoma	Blue	Orange
Ears	Indigo	Tinnitus	Magenta	Green
		Deafness	Indigo	Gold
		Ear infections	Turquoise	Red
Thyroid	Blue	Goitre	Blue	Orange
		Over-active	Blue	Orange
		Under-active	Orange	Blue
Parathyroids	Yellow	Osteoporosis	Yellow	Violet
Lungs	Green	Asthma	Blue	Orange
		Bronchitis	Orange	Blue
		Pleurisy	Blue	Orange
		Cancer	Magenta	Green
		Pneumonia	Red	Turquoise

Reflex	General reflex colour	Complaint	Colours for specific complaints	
			Treatment colour	Complementary colour
Shoulder	Blue	Frozen shoulder	Yellow	Violet
		Muscular strains or tension	Indigo	Gold
Heart	Green or rose pink	Tachycardia	Blue	Orange
		Palpitations	Blue	Orange
		Thrombosis	Magenta	Green
		Angina	Indigo	Gold
		Broken heart (emotional)	Violet/rose pink	—
Solar plexus	Yellow	Tension, stress	Blue	Orange
Gall bladder	Yellow	Stones	Orange	Blue
Liver	Yellow	Hepatitis	Indigo	Gold
		Jaundice	Blue	Orange
Stomach	Yellow	Indigestion	Yellow	Violet
		Ulcers	Blue	Orange
		Cancer	Magenta	Green
Pancreas	Yellow	Diabetes	Yellow	Violet
Kidneys	Yellow	Nephritis	Turquoise	Red
		Kidney stones	Orange	Blue
		Nephroma	Magenta	Green
		Water retention	Magenta	Green
Bladder	Green	Cystitis	Turquoise	Red
		Cancer	Magenta	Green
Small intestine	Orange	Inflammation	Indigo	Gold
		Cancer	Magenta	Green
Ileo-caecal valve	Blue	Constipation	Blue	Orange
Colon	Green	Constipation	Red	Turquoise
		Diarrhoea	Blue	Orange
		Cancer	Magenta	Green

Reflex	General reflex colour	Complaint	Colours for specific complaints	
			Treatment colour	Complementary colour
Sciatic loop	Violet	Sciatica	Indigo	Gold
Spleen	Orange	Disorders of the immune system	Turquoise	Red
		Fatigue	Orange	Blue
Ovaries	Orange	Ovarian cyst	Orange	Blue
		Pregnancy	Blue	Orange
		Infertility	Red	Turquoise
		Cancer	Magenta	Green
Uterus	Orange	Prolapse	Orange	Blue
		Pregnancy	Blue	Orange
		Tumour	Magenta	Green
		Fibroids	Orange	Blue
		Infertility	Red	Turquoise
Breast	Green	Cysts	Magenta	Green
		Cancer	Magenta	Green
		Mastitis	Blue	Orange
Lymphatic system	Turquoise	Stress	Turquoise	Red
		Any infections present	Turquoise	Red
		General treatment	Turquoise	Red
Sacroiliac joint	Yellow	Arthritis	Yellow	Violet
Prostate	Orange	Enlarged	Blue	Orange
		Cancer	Magenta	Green
Testes	Turquoise	Malignant tumour	Magenta	Green
Anus	Red	Piles	Yellow	Violet

CHAPTER 8

Helping a Person to Help Themselves with Colour

I feel that when we, as therapists, treat people with reflexology and colour, we should also instruct and help them to help themselves. Obviously, diet plays a large part in this because basically we are what we eat. The human body is a very beautiful piece of machinery which is self-repairing, given the right conditions. If we become the owner of a new car, we would make sure that it was filled with the correct petrol and oil. Likewise with our own body. If we give it the correct fuel, namely food and liquid, it will serve us well and we will be filled with energy. On the other hand, if we serve it junk food, eventually it will start to be unwell. If I feel that a patient would benefit from a change of diet, then I always refer them to a dietician.

As with diet, so a person can also help themselves with colour. Remember that we are surrounded with colour which is continually changing according to our mood and state of health. Each organ, muscle and bone in the physical body vibrates to a set frequency and therefore emanates the colour which corresponds to that frequency. If the vibrational frequency in part of the body changes, thereby causing disease, it can be amended by introducing the correct colour frequency.

Each person should be made to feel responsible for their own health and well-being, which perhaps conventional medicine is not allowing. It is so easy to visit a doctor with a set of symptoms and be given pills or medicine to take two or three times daily. This does not allow us to tune into our own body in order to find out what we have been doing which caused the disease and to subsequently rectify it so that the body can return to harmony and health. Yes, this takes effort, initiative and time, but there are no side effects and the whole process can become one of learning and evolving. By this process we are also able to help others when they have problems. It is far more beneficial to help from experience than from intellectual knowledge.

When treating with reflexology and colour, we can encourage a patient to participate in their treatment by giving them practical things to do with the colour or colours which they need. The colour needed is found through the reflexology treatment. For example, if a patient came complaining of kidney stones, orange would be recommended. If they had diabetes, it would be yellow. These colours can be found on the charts given on pages 119–21.

Some of the ways in which a patient can help themselves with colour are given below.

1. Solarized Water

For this, a glass of water is needed and a solarizer. The water solarizer is a triangular-shaped box with a stained glass top and front. The top and front are made to allow the glass to be interchangeable. It is important that stained glass is used in preference to gels for reasons already given in an earlier chapter. The address where these and other materials can be obtained is given at the back of this book.

A glass of water is placed in the solarizer with the appropriate coloured stained glass and left in the sun or daylight for three to four hours. During this time, the water becomes infused with the vibrational frequency of the colour. This water is then taken in small doses during the course of the day. For people doubting the validity of this, an interesting experiment is to solarize eight small glasses of water, each with a different colour, and then taste them. It will be found that each glass has a different taste.

2. Solarizing Quartz Crystal

Healing with crystals is a very ancient therapy, dating back to Atlantean times. The Atlanteans had large healing temples made from crystal and gemstones, for the use of people who needed healing.

Ayurvedic medicine uses crystals and gemstones which have been ground to a very fine powder and mixed with a liquid. This is then taken by the patient in the prescribed dosage. Gem remedies can also be made by boiling gems in spring water. The gem is then removed and the water further diluted to make the remedy. These methods can be time-consuming and costly, especially if one is working with precious gems.

Another way of using gems is to apply the appropriate coloured gem to the part of the body which is unwell or energy centre which is malfunctioning. For example, amethyst followed by rose quartz can be placed on the heart centre for people suffering from a 'broken' heart. Amethyst heals the wound and rose quartz fills the void which has been left with spiritual love.

A method which I have found to be very successful is to solarize quartz crystal. This is done by placing a piece of quartz crystal on top of stained glass which is placed over a lamp. This is then left for thirty minutes. The colour from the stained glass solarizes the crystal, which can then be placed on any part of the body which needs the colour.

If a person is suffering from an infected cut or graze, solarize a piece of crystal with turquoise and place this over the infection. After this has been done, the crystal should be put into salt water for twelve hours to cleanse it.

3. The Use of Coloured Silk or Cotton

For this, a piece of body-length silk approximately 6' x 2' is needed. This should be dyed with a natural dye to the colour required. (Dyes made out of natural ingredients are more harmonious to the vibrations of the physical body.) When using this, the person must be dressed completely in white or, if in the privacy of their own home, they can be naked. Lying in a warm, sunny or brightly lit room, the body is covered with the silk for twenty minutes. Because each cell of the body is light-sensitive, during this time it is able to absorb the colour. If a person suffers from hypertension, then they should lie under a piece of blue silk twice daily, preferably in the morning and last thing at night. If silk is not obtainable or too expensive to buy, then cotton can be used but it must be 100% pure cotton.

Because each cell of our body is light-sensitive, the colour of the clothes we wear also affects us. It is therefore beneficial to wear a piece of clothing in the colour which we need. Again, if it is a blouse, shirt or dress, whatever is worn underneath must be white. If we choose to wear underwear in the appropriate colour, then white must be worn on top. This is not always practical because coloured underwear will show through the white garment worn over it.

4. Colour Breathing

With this method, the colour needed is visualized and inhaled into the diseased part of the body. The red, orange and yellow rays are brought into the body through the feet, the green ray is brought in horizontally through the heart centre and the blue, turquoise, violet and magenta rays are breathed in through the top of the head. The colour is then visualized permeating the part of the body where it is required. If someone is suffering with laryngitis, then the blue ray would be visualized entering through the top of the head into the larynx. Colour breathing is also an excellent method for balancing and revitalizing the chakras.

♦ To do this, sit down in a place which is quiet and warm. Whichever position you sit in, make sure that your spine is straight. Start by relaxing the body and quieting the mind. Bring your concentration into the inhalation and exhalation of the breath. With each exhalation, breathe out any remaining tension.

On the next inhalation, visualize a shaft of pure red light entering from the earth, through your feet and into the base chakra. As you exhale, allow this colour to radiate out into your aura. This is repeated three times with each colour.

On the fourth inhalation, visualize a shaft of pure orange light entering from the earth, into your feet and into the sacral chakra. As you exhale, let it flow out into your aura. Try to feel the joy and energy that this colour brings to your body, mind and spirit.

On the seventh inhalation, bring a shaft of pure yellow light through the earth, into your feet and into the solar plexus chakra. Visualize this chakra becoming like a radiant golden sun with its energizing, healing rays touching every part of your body. Exhale and watch its pure luminous colour radiate into your aura.

On the tenth inhalation, bring a shaft of pure green light horizontally into the heart chakra. As it flows out into your aura on the exhalation, feel your body and its energies being brought into balance.

On the thirteenth inhalation, see a shaft of pure blue light enter through the top of your head, into the throat chakra. Exhaling, allow it to flow into your aura, surrounding you with a cloak of peace and tranquillity.

On the sixteenth inhalation, allow a shaft of deep indigo to enter through the top of your head, into the brow chakra. Feel it radiating out deep relaxation as it flows into your aura on the exhalation.

On the nineteenth inhalation, visualize a shaft of pure violet light entering the top of your head, into the crown chakra. As you exhale, this colour radiates into your aura and lifts upwards, changing from violet into a very pale magenta. As you look into this colour, it enables you to let go of anything which is no longer right for you. This could be old habits, conditioning, certain types of food, etc.

Sit for a while and see yourself clothed in a coat of many colours, each colour ethereal, pure and luminous. Watch as they dance around you, interweaving with each other.

When you are ready, take note of anything that you may have experienced and then start to bring yourself gently back into everyday consciousness, sealing your chakras as already described.

If you have difficulty in visualizing colour, as some people do, it can be helpful to look at a flower or some other living object which radiates the colour that you are trying to visualize. It is only with practice that the visualization of colour improves.

5. Food

The natural colour of the food which we eat can also provide us with the vibrational frequency of its colour. Therefore, if we need orange, it helps to eat food of this colour. Listed below are some foods related to the colours of the spectrum.

Red
Radishes, red cabbage, beetroot, raspberries, red cherries, red peppers, tomatoes, redcurrants, red plums

Orange
Oranges, carrots, mangoes, tangerines, pumpkins, apricots, swedes

Yellow
Yellow peppers, sweetcorn, golden plums, bananas, pineapple, cheese, parsnips, marrow, lemons, grapefruit, honeydew melons, butter and the yolk of an egg

Green
Spinach, cabbage, green peppers, watercress, lettuce, green apples, greengages, peas, green lentils and kiwi fruit

Blue
Blue plums, blueberries, grapes and bilberries

Violet
Purple grapes, purple broccoli, aubergine and plums

Magenta
Strawberries and any of the pale pink fruits and vegetables

CHAPTER 9

Case Histories

Case 1

Mr A, aged 70, came for treatment complaining of tinnitus. He said that this had started after having his ears syringed. Apparently, the first attempt at syringing had failed to remove all of the wax, thereby necessitating a further treatment. It was after the second syringing that his problems began.

I started by carrying out a normal reflexology treatment and found that the reflexes of the ears and Eustachian tubes were very painful to touch. Also the ear reflexes had crystal deposits. The solar plexus reflex was painful but I suspected that part of the cause of this was the pain that he had experienced during treatment not knowing what to expect, having never before experienced reflexology.

Having completed the treatment, I applied blue to the solar plexus through the reflexology torch. The patient started to relax and said that he felt sleepy. I then applied magenta, followed by its complementary colour green to the ear and Eustachian tube reflexes on both feet. Mr A reported that the noise in his ears started to get lower in pitch.

On his second visit, he said that the noise in his ears had heightened a little but was not so high in pitch as before his first treatment. The same treatment procedure was carried out. Again Mr A commented that the sound was becoming lower in pitch and was less loud.

Mr A attended for a further ten treatments at weekly intervals. After each treatment he noticed that the ringing in his ears was becoming quieter and lower in pitch. At the end of the last treatment, his tinnitus had almost disappeared. He said that if he became very tired he became aware of a faint noise in his ears but that it was so slight it did not unduly worry him.

Case 2

Mr B was in his late 60s and he attended complaining of blocked sinuses and a constant feeling of being deaf. I asked if he had recently had a cold, to which he replied that he had last had a cold about two months ago. Apparently, one of the effects of this cold was very bad sinusitis and this had not cleared.

Through carrying out a normal reflexology treatment, I discovered that the head, sinus and ear reflexes were very painful, especially the Eustachian tubes. At the end of the treatment, I applied indigo followed by gold to the sinus reflexes and magenta and green to the ear reflexes. I then applied red and turquoise to the sinus pressure points on the face. At the end of the treatment, Mr B said that he felt as though there was a lot of mucus becoming loose.

When he attended a week later for his second treatment, he reported that he had experienced a lot of mucus discharge and this had made his head feel clearer. The same treatment procedure was followed as the previous week. When I transmitted magenta to the ear pressure points located on the face, he said that he felt something 'pop', allowing him to be able to hear clearly again.

On his third visit, he reported further mucous discharge from his sinuses but much less than the previous week.

I gave him one further treatment and this revealed that his reflexes were much less painful. He said that he felt better, his head felt clearer and that he was again able to hear.

Case 3

Miss C, aged 24, attended complaining of insomnia, anxiety and bad circulation. Since the birth of her daughter three years previously, her menstruation had ceased. She was underweight and had been anorexic. During the counselling session prior to treatment, she said that her childhood had been very unhappy and that this had accounted for a lot of her problems as she grew up.

The initial reflexology treatment revealed the following painful reflexes: solar plexus, spinal, reproductive, splenic and kidney. After this treatment I applied blue to the solar plexus, gold to the spine, orange to the spleen and red to the reproductive organs.

On her second visit a week later, she reported a strong reaction to the previous week's treatment. She said that she had experienced very dramatic mood swings and felt that emotional blocks were being released. The previous week's treatment was repeated.

On her third visit, she informed me that she had gone through tremendous emotional distress, accompanied by vivid dreams. She said that she felt as though past experiences which she had been unable to face and had therefore buried in her unconscious were being brought into her conscious mind and these she found difficult to resolve. The same pattern of treatment was continued.

When she came the following week, she appeared much more positive in her outlook on life. We had spoken about diet and she was now eating more sensibly and had gained a little weight. After the normal reflexology treatment, when applying red to the right ovary reflex, she said that she felt that she was the child that had not been allowed to grow up. When the left ovary was treated with red, she said that she felt as though she was the adult that had not been allowed to mature. I then treated the base chakra on the spinal reflex with red and she said that she felt as though the child and the adult were merging into one. I then balanced the remaining chakras on the spinal reflex with the appropriate colours.

Miss C continued to attend for treatment for a further two months. Each week showed a gradual improvement, a new insight. When her treatment ended, she was eating sensibly, had returned to college and was able to cope with her emotional problems.

Case 4

Mrs D attended with chronic sinusitis, ear problems and chest congestion. She reported that she had undergone surgery for her sinuses and had had plastic tubes placed into both ears. After her operation, her sinuses improved for a while but were again very bad. She had been diagnosed as having a lump in her left sinus and had been advised to have it surgically removed. This she did not want to do.

During the initial reflexology treatment, the reflexes to the sinuses, ears, lungs, solar plexus and spine were very painful. Because she was experiencing so much pain, I treated these reflexes with colour; indigo and gold to the sinuses, magenta and green to the ears and chest, blue to the solar plexus and gold to the spine. I then treated the chakras on the spinal reflex with the appropriate colours.

On her second visit, she said that she had experienced a lot of mucous discharge from her sinuses and that she had developed a chesty cough. We talked about diet and she agreed to give up all dairy produce for a while, this being well known for producing mucus in the body. The previous week's treatment was repeated, using mainly colour on the reflexes which were too painful to touch.

This treatment continued on a weekly basis. On her eighth visit she reported that a soft mass had been discharged through her nose, leaving her sinuses feeling much clearer. When she subsequently returned to the hospital to have her sinuses checked, the lump which was initially diagnosed had disappeared.

Mrs D continued with her treatment for a period of six months. During this time she experienced not only tremendous improvement in her sinus and chest congestion, but also a greater sense of well-being.

Case 5

Mrs E attended complaining of pain in her lumbar spine. The pain had been with her for about six months. She had sought the advice of her doctor and had been given a course of physiotherapy. This had failed to relieve her of the pain. The only way she could mask the pain was by taking painkillers.

When carrying out the initial reflexology treatment on her feet, the spinal reflex was extremely painful. She also experienced pain in the bladder and kidney reflexes, also the solar plexus. When asked if she had had any problems with her kidneys, she said that she kept getting attacks of cystitis. I then applied turquoise to the bladder and kidney reflexes, blue to the solar plexus and indigo followed by gold to the spinal reflex. I ended the treatment by applying the relevant colours to the chakras on the spinal reflex.

When she attended for treatment the following week, she said that she had had a very bad attack of cystitis and that the pain in her back had got worse. I carried out another reflexology treatment using the same colours for the painful reflexes as the previous week.

On her third visit, she said that she felt much better and that the pain in her back seemed to be easier.

Mrs E attended for a further four treatments. The pain in her back gradually got better and finally disappeared. She then attended one month later for treatment. She said that the pain in her back had not returned, she had had no further attacks of cystitis and that she felt a completely different person.

Case 6

Mrs F was 40 and attended complaining of a lump in her right breast. She said that she had first noticed the lump whilst taking a bath. She said that she had been to her doctor who had confirmed that there was a lump. He wanted to send her to hospital in order that it could be aspirated and tested for malignancy. She had declined to do this. She had studied complementary therapies and believed that, given the right conditions, the body is self-healing.

In carrying out the initial reflexology treatment, the reflexes to the right breast, solar plexus and axillary lymph glands were very painful. I applied turquoise to the lymph glands, blue to the solar plexus and magenta followed by green to the breast reflex on both feet. I instructed the patient that twice daily she should visualize the lump encompassed in a green light that was itself surrounded by a bright white light.

Mrs F faithfully carried out her visualization exercises and attended weekly for treatment. At the end of the eighth week, she said she thought that the lump was starting to shrink, but could not be sure. By the sixteenth treatment, she reported that the lump was definitely smaller.

She continued treatment for a further three months and at the end of this time the lump had disappeared.

Case 7

Miss G was only 28 and attended with advanced cancer in both breasts. It had been diagnosed by the hospital two years earlier but she had declined to have a mastectomy. Previous to this she had had a malignant lump removed from her breast and undergone a course of radium treatment. She showed me the worst breast which was open and ulcerated where the tumour had broken through the skin. She was a lovely soul, always cheerful and positive in her outlook. I agreed to treat her but knew that the most I could do would be to try to alleviate her pain and prepare her for going into spirit.

After each reflexology treatment, I always treated the lymphatic system with turquoise, both breast reflexes with magenta and green, the solar plexus with blue, the liver with green and the spinal reflex with gold. I then applied the appropriate colours to the chakras on the spinal reflex. We talked a lot about spiritual things and what she would like to do with her life if she was healed.

When she came she said that the treatment relaxed her and took away a lot of the pain that she was experiencing, especially across her chest. Towards the end of her life, she started to talk about death and what it meant to her. It was something she did not fear. She described death as a transition.

The last time that I saw her she was still bright and cheerful and had virtually no pain. Three days after this visit she died at home surrounded by her family.

After her death, I realized that she had taught me a great deal, the most important lesson being that even if a person is terminally ill, we as therapists can help to prepare them to make the transition from this life to the next. If we can help to give them a greater sense of well-being during this time by alleviating some or all of their pain, then I think that this is a wonderful thing to do.

Case 8

Mr H attended complaining of pain in his right shoulder and cervical spine. He said that he had been suffering with it for a very long time. He was a musician by profession and played the violin. He said that the pain seemed much worse after a concert.

During the initial reflexology treatment, I found that the reflexes to the right shoulder, head and cervical spine were particularly painful. I asked him if he suffered from headaches. He said that he did and they were becoming more frequent. After I had finished the reflexology treatment, I applied blue to the head, neck, shoulder and solar plexus reflexes. I also gave him some very simple shoulder and neck exercises to do because I suspected that the main cause of his problem was tension.

When he attended the following week, he reported that his shoulder felt much easier and that he had only had one headache during the course of the week. He said that he felt that the treatment and exercises had helped him a great deal.

He attended for a further eight treatments and at the end of this time, the pain in his shoulder had gone and he had not had a headache for a month.

Case 9

Mrs I was a very nervous lady. On her first visit, she said that she had never had reflexology treatment before and that she was rather frightened, not knowing what to expect. I reassured her by explaining exactly what I was going to do. She told me that she had been through a nervous breakdown brought on by her home environment and that she had been prescribed Valium which she had been taking for the past six months. She said that she would like to come off these tablets but when she had previously tried, she had experienced severe headaches and panic attacks. I advised that she consult her doctor about this.

When carrying out the reflexology treatment, the reflexes on her feet were so painful that she would barely allow me to touch them. By the time that I had completed the first foot, she was so tense and frightened, I decided to treat just with colour through the reflexology torch.

I started by applying blue to the solar plexus reflexes. Gradually she started to relax. She said that she felt as though a warm glow of light was travelling from her feet through her body, a warm glow that made her feel very sleepy. From the solar plexus, I treated the remaining reflexes starting with the head reflex and working downwards.

As I worked on her feet with the different colours she related the various sensations that she was having. She said that the vibration of some of the colours travelled faster than others whilst other colours were only felt at particular points in the body. I found it as fascinating as she did. Unfortunately, the vibrational sensations felt when treating the lymph glands were never divulged because by this time Mrs I was fast asleep.

After I had completed the treatment, I gently woke her. She said that she felt wonderful, very relaxed and at peace with herself.

Mrs I continued treatment for three months. During this time she opened up and talked a lot about herself, her family and her home life. She also realized that there were changes which she would have to make if she was to gain a complete recovery.

Slowly, she made these changes and was able to come off Valium. The reflexes on her feet became much less painful enabling me to carry out a normal reflexology treatment before using colour.

When she attended for her last treatment, she looked a different person, more confident and positive and able to face and cope with life again.

These cases mentioned and other people whom I have treated with reflexology and colour have proved to me over and over again the value and therapeutic benefit of combining colour and reflexology.

Bibliography

Alpen, Frank, *Exploring Atlantis*, Anzona Metaphysical Society, 1981.

Bailey, Alice, *Esoteric Healing*, Lucis Trust, 1953.

Bhagavad Gita, Penguin, 1962.

Brennan, Barbara Ann, *Hands of Light*, Bantam Books, 1987.

Gimbel, Theo, *Healing Through Colour*, C.W. Daniel, 1980.

Gimbel, Theo, *Form, Sound, Colour and Healing*, C.W. Daniel, 1987.

Hunt, Ronald T., *The Seven Keys to Colour*, C.W. Daniel, 1981.

Ingham, Eunice D., *Stories the Feet Can Tell*, Ingham Publishing, 1938.

Liberman, Jacob, *Light: Medicine of the Future*, Bear & Co., 1991.

Lynes Barry, *The Healing of Cancer*, Marcus Books, 1989.

Powell, Arthur E., *The Astral Body*, The Theosophical Publishing House, 1927.

Powell, Arthur E., *The Mental Body*, The Theosophical Publishing House, 1927.

Sears, W. Gordon & Winwood, R.S., *Anatomy & Physiology for Nurses*, Edward Arnold, 1941.

St Pierre, Gaston & Boater, Debbie, *The Metamorphic Technique*, Element Books, 1982.

Tansley, David, *Radionics and the Subtle Bodies of Man*, Health Science Press, 1972.

Vivekananda, Swami, *Raja Yoga*, Advaita Ashram, 1973.

Resources

For information regarding courses pertaining to colour therapy and integrating colour with reflexology, plus information on the reflexology crystal torch and other products relating to colour therapy, contact:

Pauline Wills
The Oracle School of Colour
9 Wyndale Avenue
Kingsbury
London NW9 9PT

Tel/Fax: 0181 204 7672

Index

Tai Chi
A PRACTICAL INTRODUCTION
By Paul Crompton

Tai Chi, the Chinese art of gentle exercise, has also been described as 'meditation in movement'. Safe, effective and suitable for all ages, Tai Chi promotes excellent health and relief from stress.

In *Tai Chi: A Practical Introduction*, internationally acclaimed practitioner Paul Crompton opens the doors of this magical healing world to beginners and deepens the experience for the more advanced student. Beginning with the history and philosophy of Tai Chi he moves on to a detailed explanation of the famous Tai Chi sequence of movements, the 48 Form Set.

Illustrations, diagrams and many practical exercises will enable students of all abilities to master the basics of the ancient healing art of Tai Chi.

Paul Crompton has studied Tai Chi and martial arts for over forty years, and is an internationally recognized expert in these areas. He has written extensively on the martial arts, and his books include *The Elements of Tai Chi* and *Walking Meditation*.

ISBN 1 86204 163 6

Shiatsu
A PRACTICAL INTRODUCTION
By Oliver Cowmeadow

Developed from a traditional form of Japanese massage, Shiatsu is based upon the same philosophy and medical theory as acupuncture and other oriental healing methods. Literally translated, Shi-atsu means 'finger pressure', but practitioners also use their palms, knees and forearms, and employ stretching techniques. These combine in a simple but effective form of treatment used to promote health and general well-being, as well as to cure illness and prevent future problems.

In this straightforward step-by-step guide, Oliver Cowmeadow introduces us to the ways in which Shiatsu can be beneficial to both the person giving and the person receiving.

Shiatsu: A Practical Introduction clearly explains:
- the role of energy in Shiatsu
- how to give a full body Shiatsu treatment
- how to eat an energetically balanced diet to promote health
- how to treat simple health problems with Shiatsu
- methods of oriental diagnosis
- common uses of accupressure points
- energy balancing exercises for yourself

Oliver Cowmeadow, who has been a practitioner of Shiatsu for fourteen years, runs a successful practice in Devon and is the principal teacher and director of the Devon School of Shiatsu, running introductory and professional training courses.

'This book is a welcome contribution by one of today's mature generation of British practitioners of Shiatsu.'
NEIL GULLIVER, EAST ANGLIAN SCHOOL OF SHIATSU

ISBN 1 86204 162 8

Yoga
A PRACTICAL INTRODUCTION
Dr Svami Purna

The long-established healing regime of Hatha Yoga – the
Yoga of physical exercise – provides a complete system of
physical, mental and emotional well-being for men, women
and children, for life.

In *Yoga: A Practical Introduction*, renowned teacher
Sri Svāmi Pūrṇá leads the reader through a simple 12-week
programme. Each of the lessons revolves around a guiding
thought or principle which is manifested by related
exercises or postures. Breathing and relaxation techniques,
dietary advice, and aids to concentration and meditation are
also included.

Sri Svāmi Pūrṇá was born into an Indian family of
philosophers and rulers. He is a Sanskrit master and a doctor
of medicine, psychology and literature, and his mastery of
the six schools of Indian philosophy and the Eightfold Path
of Yoga have earned him worldwide recognition and the title
Vidya Vacaspati, Lord of Learning.

ISBN 1 86204 164 4